P9-CSB-516

QUALITY IMPROVEMENT IN WOMEN'S HEALTH CARE

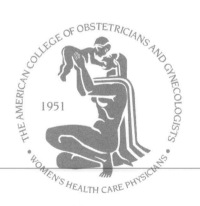

The American College
of Obstetricians and
Gynecologists
Women's Health Care Physicians

Committee on Quality Assessment (1999–2000)
Anthony L. Angello, MD, *Chairman*
James F. Blute III, MD, *Vice Chairman*
Mark D. Pearlman, MD
Richard C. Pees, MD
Michael R. Tesoro, MD
Angela R. Watson, RN
Michael P. Woods, MD

Special thanks also are extended to Paul A. Gluck, MD; Johanna F. Perlmutter, MD; and Carol W. Saffold, MD, former members of the Committee on Quality Assessment, and to Ann Allen, JD, former staff member.

Staff
Stanley Zinberg, MD, MS, *Vice President, Division of Practice Activities*
Penny Rutledge, JD, *General Counsel*
Pamela K. Scarrow, CPHQ, *Manager, Quality Assessment*
LaShawn C. Jordan, *VRQC Administrator*
Adrienne D. Ali, *Administrative Assistant*

Clinical opinions expressed herein are based on a variety of ACOG publications. They are neither comprehensive in scope nor exhaustive in detail but rather are designed to provide general guidelines. The Committee encourages the use of this manual as a resource in developing local criteria.

Library of Congress Cataloging-in-Publication Data

Quality improvement in women's health care.
      p. ; cm.
   Prepared by the Committee on Quality Assessment of the American College of Obstetricians and Gynecologists.
   Rev. ed. of: Quality assessment and improvement in obstetrics and gynecology. 1994 ed.
   Includes bibliographical references.
   ISBN 0-915473-63-1 (pbk. : alk. paper)
   1. Gynecology—Quality control. 2. Obstetrics—Quality control. 3. Gynecology—United States—Quality control. 4. Obstetrics—United States—Quality control. I. American College of Obstetricians and Gynecologists. Committee on Quality Assessment. II. Quality assessment and improvement in obstetrics and gynecology.
   [DNLM: 1. Obstetrics—standards—United States. 2. Gynecology—standards—United States. 3. Quality Assurance, Health Care—methods—United States. WQ 100 Q15 2000]
RG103.4 .Q354 2000
618'.068'5—dc21

                              00-045409

Copyright © 2000 by the American College of Obstetricians and Gynecologists, 409 12th Street, SW, PO Box 96920, Washington, DC 20090-6920

2345/10987

CONTENTS

PREFACE

In 1994, the American College of Obstetricians and Gynecologists (ACOG) published *Quality Assessment and Improvement in Obstetrics and Gynecology*, which joined a long line of publications developed by ACOG to inform and assist Fellows who participate in peer review and quality improvement activities. This revision, *Quality Improvement in Women's Health Care,* is intended to serve as a primer for obstetricians and gynecologists starting or managing quality improvement programs within their respective hospitals. Some information may be adapted for use in the ambulatory setting.

The manual is divided into three parts: Part 1 provides an overview of quality assessment activities as they currently exist in the United States, followed by information on the specific steps involved in establishing and maintaining a quality improvement program. Part 2 addresses the issue of assessing clinical competence, one of the key elements of any quality improvement program and certainly a major responsibility for ob-gyn department chairpersons. Finally, Part 3 contains ACOG Screening Tools, which can be used for retrospective chart review to evaluate the quality of patient care. Together, these three sections provide sufficient information to enable a newly appointed department chairperson to embark on a quality improvement program.

QUALITY IMPROVEMENT
IN WOMEN'S HEALTH CARE

PART 1

DEVELOPING A DEPARTMENTAL QUALITY IMPROVEMENT PROGRAM

BACKGROUND

The Institute of Medicine (IOM), in its 1990 report *Medicare: A Strategy for Quality Assurance*, defined quality of care as "the degree to which health services for individuals and populations increase the likelihood of desired health outcomes and are consistent with current professional qualities" (1). The process by which the health care evaluation is performed has changed over the years; however, the ultimate goal remains the same—to improve the overall quality of care provided to all patients, including "improving the patient–customer experience" (2).

The Joint Commission on Accreditation of Healthcare Organizations (referred to as the Joint Commission) initially made only general references to assessing and improving care. In 1975, the Quality of Professional Services standard was published. It required hospitals to "demonstrate that the quality of patient care was consistently optimal by continually evaluating care through reliable and valid measures," mostly through time-limited audits of care. In 1985, the Joint Commission replaced the problem-focused approach with a requirement for systematic monitoring and evaluation of important aspects of patient care. The Joint Commission then began developing its now-well-known 10-step monitoring and evaluation process (3). This model was extensively discussed in ACOG's 1994 publication, *Quality Assessment and Improvement in Obstetrics and Gynecology*.

The traditional quality assurance model focused primarily on untoward events and problem physicians rather than process and system failures. This model identified outliers and the associated resources used, but was directed at only those 10% of people or outcomes that fell outside a given threshold. There was no action or education for the 90% of people or outcomes that fell within the threshold (3).

In 1989, Donald M. Berwick, MD, wrote the landmark column on continuous improvement as an ideal in health care. In this article, Dr. Berwick discussed the "Theory of Bad Apples," espoused by many at the time. To achieve quality, they asserted, required removing physicians who practiced substandard care (ie, the "bad apples"). The Theory of Bad Apples was geared toward a punitive rather than an educational approach. He suggested that what was needed instead was continuous improvement. W. Edwards Deming and Joseph M. Juran had discovered that problems, and therefore opportunities to improve quality, usually are process based. Consequently, the focus should be on continuous improvement to reduce waste, rework, and complexity (4).

Another leader in health care quality, Avedis Donabedian, MD, MPH, articulated what continues to serve as the unifying conceptual framework for quality measurement and assurance. Dr. Donabedian defined quality as a difficult-to-identify property that medical care has in varying degrees and which, even if identified, requires translation into criteria and standards that can be used in making consistent judgments. He divided the concept of patient management into technical care, which is the application of science and technology of medicine, and interpersonal care, which is the management of the social and psychologic interactions between physician and patient (5). Even more important, his widely accepted model of structure, process, and outcome has guided more than two decades of research and program development (6). *Structure* includes the resources associated with the provision of care (staffing, equipment, space). *Process* activities analyze the practice of care delivery through direct observation of patient care and studies based on the medical record. Finally, *outcomes* studies emphasize the results of care and intervention of the health care provider. Essentially, this three-part approach is possible only because good structure increases the likelihood of good process, and good process increases the likelihood of a good outcome (7).

Over the years, the focus of quality improvement efforts has shifted from a punitive approach to an educational one. The quality improvement process assists all providers at all levels of care. Therefore, the ongoing monitoring and evaluation of clinical patient care should be implemented through a process known as *continuous quality improvement* (CQI). This section describes in detail the steps necessary to develop a program to monitor the quality of care in a typical hospital department of obstetrics and gynecology. Portions of this process may apply to the ambulatory setting. Although a number of different terms are used for this process (quality assessment, quality management, performance improvement), for purposes of this document, the term *quality improvement* (QI) will be used.

GETTING ORGANIZED

According to the authors of *Guide to Clinical Resource Management*, "the first and most important responsibility of a quality and utilization management department is to provide leadership for the development, implementation, and coordination of the organization's plan to improve organizational performance" (8). In hospitals, medical staff leadership roles and responsibilities vary depending on the organizational structure of the institution. Three institutional models are common:

1. Community hospitals with a voluntary medical staff

2. Hospitals with a closed medical staff (with or without salaried physicians)

3. Academic centers with medical staffs composed of a mixture of physicians employed by the medical school, hospital, or department, as well as physicians who have private practices or are voluntary, community-based physicians, or both (9)

Regardless of the structure within a given hospital, responsive leadership in the department of obstetrics and gynecology, with support from the chief executive officer, the medical executive committee, and the governing board, is key to an effective ob-gyn QI program and to the overall operation of the department.

Effective department leadership also is critical for spearheading and initiating CQI activities. It is the foundation for an effective program, providing support, funding, and resources. Strong leadership will be extremely helpful in soliciting buy-in from physicians and others within the ob-gyn department. Cooperation of departmental members will help minimize obstacles.

DEVELOPING TOOLS

According to the Joint Commission, "performance is *what* is done and *how well* it is done to provide health care. Characteristics of *what* is done and *how well* it is done are called *dimensions of performance:*

- Doing the right thing (efficacy and appropriateness), and

- Doing the right thing well (availability, timeliness, effectiveness, continuity, safety, efficiency, and respect and caring)" (10).

The following tools are useful in assessing quality and determining overall performance.

Clinical Pathways

Although the definition of clinical pathways may vary, simply stated, they are plans for the provision of clinical services that have expected time frames and resources targeted to specific diagnoses or procedures. Clinical pathways frequently are developed for high-volume, resource-intensive, and costly procedures. They are interdisciplinary, merging the medical and nursing plans of care with those of other disciplines, such as physical therapy, nutrition, and mental health. Clinical pathways are not standards of care, but rather serve as reminders of those interventions the health care team believes most likely to be needed by the "average" patient. Deviations from a pathway are to be expected; however, rationale for the deviation must be documented in the medical record. Clinical pathways can be particularly useful as a framework for outcomes management activities. (For a sample clinical pathway, see Figure 1.) A clinical pathway development process,

This example is provided for educational purposes only. It may require modification for use in a particular facility.

Outcome: Comfort is achieved with oral pain medication. Bowel and bladder function is normal. Patient is coping with change in body image. Infection is absent.

Date or Time					
Time Frame	**Preadmission Test**	**Day of or Preoperative**	**Postoperative 0–12 hours**	**12–24 hours**	**24 hours +**
Assessments and evaluations		Nsg. database completed Nsg. assessment Vital signs	Routine vital signs every 1/2 h for 2 h, then every 1 h for 4 h, then every 4 h Nsg. assessment	Vital signs every 4 h Nsg. assessment	Nsg. assessment Vital signs every 4 h
Consults		Anesthesiology			
Diagnostics	Lab per MD CXR per MD ECG per MD	All results on chart		CBC	
Diet/fluid balance		NPO IV started	IV fluids as ordered Clear liquids Catheter output I&O	I&O Saline lock IV Regular diet	I&O Regular diet
Activity/safety		Bed rails up	Bed rails up Ambulatory with assist when FC removed, then 4 times daily	Ambulatory with assistance as desired	Up as desired
Education	Hysterectomy book Self-catheter-ization instruction	Preop/Postop teaching Obtain permits Preop meds	TCDB Postop Care Reinforce pathway with patient/family *Address psychosocial needs (*Document IPR Form)	Activity levels Nutrition Hygiene Hysterectomy booklet given if not provided preoperatively	
Medication		Preop meds if ordered	PCA pump IM meds Oral pain meds Antiemetics	Oral pain meds Stool softeners Home meds	Stool softeners Oral pain meds Home meds
Treatment modalities			TCDB every 2 h Remove vaginal pack Remove catheter 8 h postop		
Discharge planning		Initiate D/C planning	Home health consult if ordered	D/C sheets completed and signed by MD	D/C sheets completed and signed per patient

*This protocol is a general guideline and does not represent a professional care standard governing providers' obligations to patients. Care is indi-vidualized to meet patients need.

Abbreviations: Nsg indicates nursing; Lab, laboratory tests; CXR, chest X-ray; ECG, electrocardiogram; MD, physician; CBC, complete blood count; NPO, nothing by mouth; IV, intravenous; I&O, input and output; FC, Foley catheter; preop, preoperative; postop, postoperative; meds, medica-tion; TCDB, turn, cough, and deep breathe; IPR, interpersonal relationships; PCA, patient-controlled analgesia; D/C, discharge.

Fig. 1. Sample Clinical Pathway: Vaginal Hysterectomy (Courtesy of Angela R. Watson, RN, Baptist Health Systems)

developed by the Dartmouth–Hitchcock Medical Center (11), includes the following steps:

1. Define population.
2. Identify pathway aim.
3. Select work group.
4. Identify measures of pathway success.
5. Create a flowchart of the steps and outcomes of current process of care and treatment of this patient population.
6. Identify areas of internal variability.
    6a. Compare to and analyze steps and outcomes of external practice(s).
7. Develop "best" practice (pathway of patient care).
8. Define specific changes to achieve optimal practice.
9. Identify format.
10. Define criteria for progression to achieve outcomes and identify potential variances.
11. Define practice steps required to achieve identified outcomes.
12. Validate or revise document with other process owners.
13. Develop instructions for use.
14. Develop implementation and an in-service plan for trial.
15. Implement trial.
16. Evaluate trial.
17. Review document and instructions for use.
18. Implement.
19. Develop and implement maintenance and enhancement plan.

Quality Indicators

A quality indicator is a measurable dimension (eg, a medical event, procedure, diagnosis, or outcome) that is considered an important aspect of care. It is not a direct measure of quality, only a tool to assess performance. Thus, an indicator can provide an assessment of the performance data of an organization or a practitioner. An indicator can be a structure (eg, a resource), a process (eg, an event or activity), or an outcome of a process or of patient health about which data are collected during monitoring activities. Examples of process and outcome indicators are shown in Table 1.

Most of the sample clinical indicators included in Table 2 are generic screens. That is, they are general elements of medical–surgical care and patient outcome that can be extracted easily from medical records to identify those cases that may require peer review to determine whether medical care was appropriate. Each

Table 1. Examples of Process and Outcome Indicators

	Outcomes	Processes
Clinical	Adverse drug reactions	Patient examination
	Patient satisfaction	Medication administration
	Readmission within 72 hours of discharge for same problem	Meal tray preparation and delivery
	Maternal mortality	Patient/family education
Organizational	Regulatory body citation	Product selection
	Delayed discharge	Preventive maintenance
	Procedure delay	Results reporting
	Staff turnover rate/vacancies	Patient registration
		Sequence of test scheduling
		Recruitment procedures

Reprinted/adapted with permission from Kazandjian VA, Sternberg EL. The epidemiology of quality. Gaithersburg, Maryland: Aspen Publishers, ©1995:128, Exhibit 8-1

TABLE 2. Sample Clinical Indicators

Obstetric Clinical Indicators	Gynecologic Clinical Indicators
A. Maternal Indicators	1. Unplanned readmission within 14 days
1. Maternal mortality	2. Admission after a return visit to the emergency room for the same problem
2. Unplanned maternal readmission within 14 days	3. Cardiopulmonary arrest, resuscitated
3. Maternal cardiopulmonary arrest, resuscitated	4. Occurrence of an infection not present on admission
4. In-hospital initiation of antibiotics 24 hours or more following term vaginal delivery	5. Unplanned admission to special (intensive) care unit
5. Unplanned removal, injury, or repair of organ during operative procedure	6. Unplanned return to operating room for surgery during the same admission
6. Excessive maternal blood loss	7. Ambulatory surgery patient admitted or retained for complication of surgery or anesthesia
a. Required transfusion	8. Gynecologic surgery, except radical hysterectomy or exenteration, using 2 or more units of blood, or postoperative hematocrit of less than 24% or hemoglobin of less than 8 g
b. Postpartum anemia hematocrit less than 22%, hemoglobin less than 7 g (decline of antepartum hematocrit of 11% or hemoglobin decline of 3.5 g)	9. Unplanned removal, injury, or repair of organ during operative procedure
7. Maternal length of stay in excess of 1 day greater than the local standard after vaginal or cesarean delivery	10. Initiation of antibiotics more than 24 hours after surgery
8. Eclampsia	11. Discrepancy between preoperative diagnosis and postoperative tissue report
9. Delivery unattended by the "responsible" physician*	12. Removal of uterus weighing less than 280 g for leiomyomata
10. Unplanned postpartum return to delivery room or operating room for management	13. Removal of follicular cyst or corpus luteum of ovary
11. Cesarean delivery for uncertain fetal status	14. Hysterectomy performed on woman younger than 30 years except for malignancy
12. Cesarean delivery for failure to progress	15. Gynecologic death
B. Neonatal Indicators	
13. Deaths of infants weighing 500 g or more subcategorized by intrahospital neonatal deaths, total stillborns, and intrapartum stillborns	
14. Delivery of an infant at less than 32 weeks of gestation in an institution without a neonatal intensive care unit	
15. Transfer of a neonate to a neonatal intensive care unit in another institution.	

*To be defined by each institution

department should formulate a list of clinical indicators, selecting those that cover a broad range of activities and address the important aspects of care provided by the department.

Indicators may be monitors of sentinel events, such as maternal death (Table 2, obstetric clinical indicator A1), where every case should be reviewed, frequently on an expedited basis. They may monitor specific rates, such as with excess blood loss (Table 2, obstetric clinical indicator A6). If the frequency of a rate-based indicator exceeds the departmental threshold or changes in frequency over time, an in-depth review may be needed. Indicators may be positive and desirable, such as detection and treatment of chlamydia, or negative, such as an unplanned return to the operating room (Table 2, gynecologic clinical indicator 6). The Joint Commission outlines components of quality that should be considered as a department develops its own set of indicators as shown in the box.

Indicators should be defined so that they can be benchmarked and the results compared with regional or national norms. Risk adjustment methods should be used when possible. Deviations from the norm can then be readily identified. Physician profiles also may be developed so that an individual's practice pattern for each indicator can be compared with department and national or regional benchmarks. For example, if the department detects an increase in the number of charts flagged for the indicator "Gynecologic surgery, except radical hysterectomy or exenteration, using 2 or more units of blood, or postoperative hematocrit of less than 24% or hemoglobin of less than 8 g" (Table 2 gynecologic clinical indicator 8) and an investigation of the cases indicates that most were hysterectomies performed by the two physicians, a review of the surgical techniques and indications for surgery used by the two physicians would be appropriate. Such profiles will form part of the database used to make decisions on granting or renewing clinical privileges and can be used to show improvement over time. Such deviations from the norm do not necessarily indicate inappropriate care. Use of a clinical indicator may flag cases managed by a particular physician which, when peer reviewed, appear to show plausible reasons for the variations. However, continued monitoring over time (referred to as *trending*) may demonstrate that this physician has a much higher rate of variation than the department as a whole. Therefore, trending data may suggest a problem, such as surgical technique, that an individual case review does not identify.

Components of Quality

Accessibility of care: The ease with which patients can obtain the care they need when they need it

Appropriateness of care: The degree to which the correct care is provided, given the current state of knowledge

Continuity of care: The degree to which the care needed by patients is coordinated among practitioners and across organizations and time

Effectiveness of care: The degree to which care is provided in the correct manner—ie, without error, given the current state of knowledge

Efficacy of care: The degree to which a service has the potential to meet the need for which it is used

Efficiency of care: The degree to which the care received has the desired effect with a minimum of effort, expense, or waste

Patient-perspective issues: The degree to which patients and their families are involved in the decision-making processes in matters pertaining to their health, and the degree to which they judge care to be acceptable.

Safety of the care environment: The degree to which the environment is free from hazard or danger.

Timeliness of care: The degree to which care is provided to patients when they need it.

©Joint Commission on Accreditation of Healthcare Organizations. Development and application of indicators for continuous improvement in prenatal care. Oakbrook Terrace, Illinois: JCAHO, 1992:18. Reprinted with permission.

Institutions may wish to define acceptable levels of care for different indicators (ie, thresholds). A *threshold* is a data point that, when reached or crossed, signals an outlier that needs further investigation and evaluation. Using thresholds is a method for deciding when an issue should be addressed and where first to look for possible problems without requiring peer review of all records. The threshold level chosen as the standard for the institution should be supported by the best available clinical and QI literature. Information on local and national rates of complications may be obtained from the respective state health data organization, the

National Center for Health Statistics, or the Agency for Healthcare Research and Quality (AHRQ). Thresholds may need to be changed as new technology evolves and treatments improve.

Standards, Guidelines, and Criteria

To measure and evaluate quality of care, it is helpful to compare it with some acceptable standard. Each department needs to develop basic guidelines about what should and should not be done in the diagnosis and management of obstetric and gynecologic conditions.

Much has been written in the literature about the development of practice guidelines, quality review criteria, and clinical protocols. The American College of Obstetricians and Gynecologists publishes guidelines as Practice Bulletins that are categorized according to the strength of the scientific evidence to support them. The College also has produced Screening Tools for use by nonphysician reviewers to aid in identifying practice variances that might indicate the need for further review, documentation, or justification (see Part 3). Only peer review can determine whether such variances are appropriate.

A department may develop its own screening tools or rely on tools developed by other organizations, including ACOG. Criteria pertaining to patient care should be selected, developed, and adapted by experts in the particular clinical area. Once drafted, these documents should be reviewed and approved by members of the department. This process will greatly improve compliance and acceptance of the criteria during implementation. Periodically, these criteria should be reviewed and either revised, reaffirmed, or withdrawn.

In *Using Clinical Practice Guidelines to Evaluate Quality of Care*, the Agency for Health Care Policy and Research (now AHRQ) distinguished the terms *guidelines, criteria, measure,* and *standard*, with examples of each, as shown in the box (12).

Regardless of the tools used, buy-in must be obtained from the leadership (administration, physician, nursing) before development and implementation of these tools can be successful. The following suggestions may be useful in gaining physician buy-in for practice guidelines (13):

1. Identify guidelines that address areas of clinical importance to physicians.
2. Establish guideline credibility.
3. Customize guidelines with physician involvement.

Example of a Clinical Practice Guideline–Derived Evaluation Tool for Determining Quality of Care for Postoperative Pain Control

Clinical practice guideline recommendations: Pain should be assessed and documented routinely at regular intervals postoperatively, as determined by the operation and the severity of pain (eg, every 2 hours while awake for 24 hours after surgery).

Medical review criterion: For the patient recovering from surgery, the patient's pain was assessed and documented every 2 hours while awake for the first 24 hours following surgery.

Performance measure: Calculate the following for consecutive surgical patients seen over a 6-month period: the number of patients whose pain was assessed and documented every 2 hours while awake. The performance measure is:

$$\frac{\text{number of cases with criterion met}}{\text{number of surgery cases}} \times 100\%$$

Standard of quality: A performance rate of 95% or less triggers a review to determine how to improve assessing and documenting the patient's pain status every 2 hours while awake for the first 24 hours postoperatively.

---

4. Break guidelines down into their simplest and most important components; key in on decision points.
5. Target the audience, to reach only those people necessary to put a guideline in practice.
6. Enlist physician champions to promote your guidelines.
7. Make it easy for physicians to follow guidelines.
8. Allocate the resources necessary to support guideline recommendations.
9. Make quality—not compliance—the basis for physician accountability.
10. Measure improvement and share the data.
11. Keep guidelines relevant by updating them.
12. Align financial incentives with quality improvement goals.

QUALITY IMPROVEMENT MODEL

Quality measurement should determine whether the processes of care provided to a single patient or population of patients 1) achieved good outcomes (outcomes measurement) or 2) represented those processes that are thought or known to be associated with achievement of good outcomes (process measurement) (12).

At the heart of quality improvement methodology is what has been referred to as the quality management cycle or the Shewhart cycle: Plan–Do–Check–Act (PDCA). A variation of this model, Plan–Do–Study–Act, has been used as a framework for accelerating improvement in a variety of business contexts (Fig. 2).

IMPLEMENTATION

This section describes the steps necessary to develop a program for continuously improving the quality of care in a typical hospital department of obstetrics and gynecology. Portions of this process also may apply to the ambulatory setting.

Leadership

Leadership has been defined as "a set of processes that creates organizations in the first place or adapts them to significantly changing circumstances. Leaders define what the future should look like, align people with that vision, and inspire them to make it happen despite the obstacles" (14).

The establishment of effective leadership is essential in developing a QI program. The chair of the department ultimately is responsible for QI activities. When physicians accept these leadership positions, their primary purpose is to establish an environment in which quality improvements can thrive.

A departmental QI committee may include the following members, with consideration given to the vice chair of the department serving as the committee chair:

- Representative physicians with varying levels of clinical experience (junior and senior staff) within the department
- Representative subspecialists, when available
- House staff member, when appropriate
- The department chair (ex officio)

The rules and regulations of the department should outline the responsibilities of the QI committee and provide information on committee size, term of office, and method of appointment. Meeting guidelines also

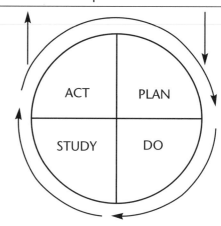

The three fundamental questions can be addressed in any order. The Plan–Do–Study–Act (PDSA) cycle is used to test and implement changes in real work settings.

PLAN: State the objectives of the cycle.
Make predictions about what will happen and why.
Develop a plan to carry out the change (Who? What? Where? What data need to be collected?).

DO: Carry out the test.
Document problems and unexpected observations.
Begin analysis of the data.

STUDY   Complete the analysis of the data.
Summarize what was learned.

ACT: What modifications should be made?
What will happen in the next cycle?

Fig. 2. Plan–Do–Study–Act Cycle (Langley GJ, Nolan KM, Nolan TW, Norman CL, Provost LP. The improvement guide: a practical approach to enhancing organizational performance. Copyright © 1996. Reprinted by permission of Jossey-Bass, Inc., a subsidiary of John Wiley & Sons, Inc.)

should be established. Part of the role of this committee and the department chair is to create an atmosphere whereby providers are able to raise quality issues in a confidential manner. Monthly meetings often are most productive and allow concurrent and retrospective case analysis.

The QI process should involve participation of all practitioners providing care at the hospital, group, and private practice levels. Participants in case reviews must be sensitive to potential conflicts of interest and scrupulously adhere to a consistent and unbiased process. When appropriate, physicians, including those from other specialties, physician assistants, certified nurse-midwives, nurse practitioners, registered nurses, and social workers may need to form a multidisciplinary task force to address specific issues that surface during the QI review process. At all times, confidentiality must be maintained. Minutes of previous meetings at which peer review activities are documented should be circulated only during the meetings themselves.

Screening Medical Records

Accurate and thorough collection of data allows identification of cases at variance with established standards and, ultimately, determination of the quality of care provided. Chart analysis following discharge seems to be the most accurate method of data retrieval. Although charts may be reviewed on a concurrent or a retrospective basis, retrospective chart review is more commonly used for screening medical records for quality review purposes. Using quality indicators or screening criteria, a trained data abstractor should screen all charts of patients discharged from the department of obstetrics and gynecology to identify cases that require further assessment by the department's QI committee. A member of the hospital QI department or department of medical records generally is responsible for the abstraction process.

The medical records department should be asked to place the records for all patients discharged from the department of obstetrics and gynecology in a single location each day, as soon after discharge as the basic information is complete. For obstetric patients, it is essential that the maternal and infant records be placed together if they are discharged on the same day. Fetal monitor records, when available, should be included as part of this process.

For efficiency, the abstractor should collect pertinent data daily. Collecting data on a regular basis ensures that the number of records will be manageable and that only a short time will be needed to complete the task. The abstractor must be familiar with medical records, medical terminology, and, ideally, the specialties of obstetrics and gynecology. Experience has shown that abstractors familiar with the system can collect the necessary data from both the maternal and infant records in less than 5 minutes.

When data analysis shows that care provided meets preestablished criteria or that performance goals have been met, the satisfactory performance should be recorded and the monitoring and evaluation system should continue. These results should be communicated to the entire staff. Parameters to help achieve performance improvement goals should be recorded, shared with all personnel, and used to improve the standards of the department. Such positive feedback and reinforcement emphasizes the philosophy that the goal of the program is higher achievement, not punitive action.

When patients' records are flagged as outliers, the abstractor should indicate the reason for flagging the record. This information can be tracked for each physician for peer review, trending, and feedback. Any records identified as varying significantly from the threshold should be referred to the QI committee for further chart review. When the data for a month have been recorded, the data collection forms are given to the individual responsible for QI activity in the department. In some institutions, the data are entered into a computer, where they can be used to generate a variety of reports. Samples of formats for department- and practitioner-specific data summaries are included in Appendixes A and B.

Either a manual system or a computer program may be used to document the results of this record review. Data reports can be generated more easily and more directly if a computer program is used, but such an aid is not essential.

Another QI process involves the acquisition of information and concerns from hospital sources outside the obstetrics and gynecology department. These sources include the nursing department and hospital committees such as those concerned with surgical review (tissue and nontissue), infection control, use of blood and blood products, and medication use. Reports from such sources may identify a problem that requires evaluation of the department as a whole or a focused review of an individual's practice. For example, the tissue committee may identify an increase in the number of small uteri removed for fibroids, prompting the department to review charts of all hysterectomies for this indication.

The Screening Tool on hysterectomy for leiomyomata (see Part 3) would be useful in such a review.

Medical Record Review

Once a case fails to meet preestablished criteria, a chart review should occur. Chart review is an objective evaluation of the case as documented in the patient's medical record. The cases identified for review in a particular month should be divided equally among the committee members with a primary reviewer assigned to each case. Cases may be referred to a generalist physician for review; however, if that review renders an adverse opinion, it should be referred to a subspecialist for review, as appropriate. The physician reviewer is responsible for reviewing the chart and determining the adequacy of care according to published guidelines, institutional clinical protocols, technical or educational bulletins, or other sources. Deviations from "norms" (ie, guidelines, protocols, criteria sets, and policy statements) may be acceptable variations or actually may be deficiencies. When deviations occur, the rationale should be documented in the medical record.

Care must be taken to ensure confidentiality in the review process. A signed copy of the hospital's confidentiality statement should be maintained. Although it may be ideal for cases not to be reviewed by direct competitors or by physicians in the same practice as the person being reviewed, this is not always practical. The possibility of bias should be considered in evaluating the results of such reviews. *Any provider who may have a conflict of interest or has participated in the care of the individual should not participate in the evaluation process.* Problems also may be identified through one of the following mechanisms:

- Provider-raised issues. The QI committee must create an atmosphere that encourages all providers to refer cases of concern and ensure that all quality issues will be handled in a confidential manner.

- Use of clinical indicators (refer to Table 2 for clinical indicators). Using Physicians' Current Procedural Terminology (CPT) and International Classification of Diseases, Ninth Revision, Clinical Modification (ICD-9-CM) codes for the indicators may facilitate the selection process.

- Referral of cases from sources outside the department, including risk management, patients or family members, other health facilities, insurance carriers, ancillary services, and information referred from the state medical board or other regulatory agency.

The primary reviewer should prepare a summary of the case to be presented and discussed at the next QI committee meeting. A consensus of opinion by the committee regarding the case must then follow. Categories of decision on a chart review might include:

A. No deficiencies found—care appropriate. Morbidity occurred despite appropriate and timely therapy.

B. Opportunity for improvement

1. Insufficient documentation of care

2. Incomplete preoperative evaluation or prenatal care

3. Inappropriate care

   a. Attending physician

   b. House staff

4. System deficiencies

   a. Nursing

   b. Ancillary services

   c. Other departments (eg, pathology, anesthesiology)

   d. Administration

It is necessary to maintain a record of all actions reviewed to identify trends that are collectively important, even though the care provided in individual cases may not have been judged to be substandard or to require corrective action. Both institutional and individual databases can thereby be developed. These data can then be compared with regional and national thresholds, when available, to determine the relative quality of care in the department.

Patterns identified by trending can reveal much about the appropriateness of care. Practice variations and deficiencies, including complications associated with them, become obvious when similar types of cases are reviewed over a period of time and across all providers. For example, insufficient justification for surgery becomes a valid measure of the appropriateness of care, especially when analysis identifies one physician performing a number of such procedures. If trending reveals a pattern within the department, such as a high postoperative infection rate, the department chair may initiate a program targeted to correct the problem.

The department also may wish to establish thresholds, defining levels of care for different indicators.

Institutions should define acceptable quality by determining their own thresholds (ie, the acceptable rate of occurrence for rate-based indicators). Thresholds may be based on data from the literature or on national averages when available. They also may be derived locally through the use of statistical control charts that document local experience. Thresholds may need to be changed as new technology evolves and treatments improve.

A well-designed and well-implemented QI program will prove effective in clearly identifying problems in care. Some acceptable variations are found during the peer review process where no action is necessary.

Following the evaluation of charts from the outliers, those variations that represent inadequate judgment, skill, or performance should be classified as deficiencies in care. When a deficiency in care is identified, there is a problem that must be corrected. When the quality of care is acceptable but could be better, there is an opportunity for improvement. Figure 3 illustrates a sample chart review process.

Quality Improvement Projects

It is important to recognize that most ob-gyns are dedicated to providing the best care possible for their patients. Continuous quality improvement should be a continuous process to improve the health care of women while at the same time providing education to physicians. Deficiencies are more likely to result from lack of information or documentation than from improper management. Therefore, a strong departmental focus on education enhances quality of care and should correct most deficiencies that are identified. The QI committee should look at trends in care within the department and identify those areas that need improvement. When adverse outcomes increase, the source of this change should be identified. One should look to see if there is a clustering of events—the hour of the day, new instruments, new staff, new procedures, or an individual provider or other personnel. Current data can be compared through statistical analysis with previous years and with national statistics. This will target those areas that need improvement.

Once strong leadership has been established, the next step, based on the data collected, is to select a QI project of a process that is creating ongoing problems for others in the process (15). The key to project selection is to have data support a topic that is not too large in scope and can be solved in a reasonable amount of time. Data should provide information about the system, not individuals or departments. The scientific method can be used to define problems by stating questions, making a plan, formulating hypotheses, gathering data to test those hypotheses, drawing conclusions, and testing those conclusions. For a sample QI project, see Table 3.

A project is more likely to succeed if the issue occurs frequently and involves substantial cost, evidence of variation in practice exists, and data are easily available. Other criteria for selecting good improvement projects include the following:

- Choosing processes that managers and employees believe need to be improved
- Choosing processes that are clearly defined—those with clear starting and ending points
- Choosing processes that have short "cycle times," so that data are readily available and the effects of interventions are easier to study
- Avoiding working on processes for which change is currently planned or already underway

When the project is identified, "opportunity statements" should be prepared for use by the team. These statements should not mention causes or remedies, should define problems and processes of manageable size, and should mention measurable characteristics, if possible (16).

At this point in the process, it is very important to obtain physician support; otherwise, the success of the project may be impeded. One of the best ways to bring physicians on board with quality improvement projects is to capitalize on their scientific training. Many physicians work well with data and tend to respond positively when given evidence supporting a project (17).

Creating Teams

For the quality improvement project selected, a team should be chosen to include representatives from all affected services and areas to ensure that all the key stakeholders in the process are involved. By quantifying the problem and stratifying the data, one can invite the most appropriate people to join the team.

A manager or other leader who has partial or complete responsibility for the process being studied should be designated team leader. This person should be in a position to remove obstacles encountered by the team. Another key team member is a facilitator who can

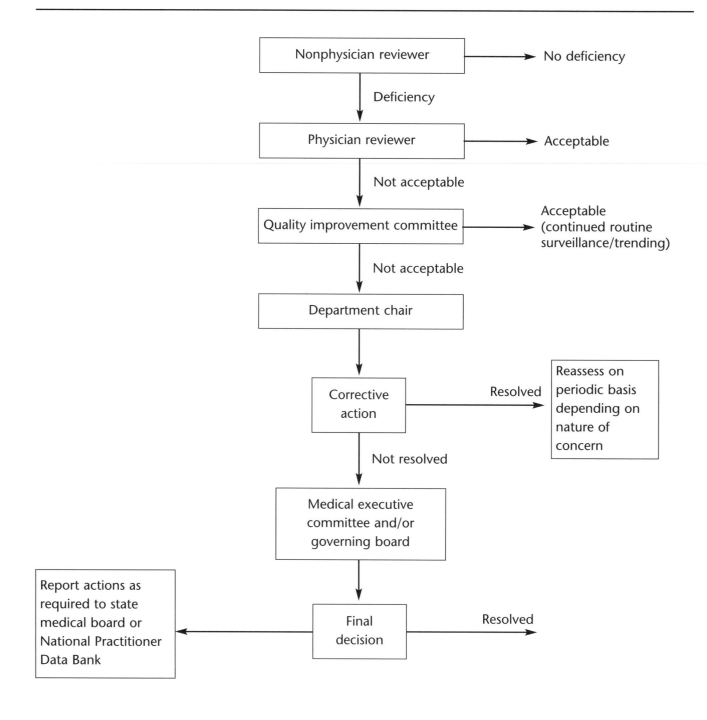

Fig. 3. Sample Chart Review Process

Table 3. Sample Quality Improvement Project: Improving care for maternity patients

Topic	Sample Measures
A. Reducing cesarean rates, when appropriate, while maintaining or improving maternal and newborn outcomes	Total cesarean rate VBAC* rates Primary cesarean rate Repeat cesarean rate Apgar scores Other maternal and neonatal morbidity and mortality measures Patient satisfaction scores
B. Improving patient experience of care throughout prenatal care and delivery, and after discharge	Patient satisfaction survey scores: • Pain management • Knowledge of care of infant after discharge • Physicians' and nurses' answers to questions understood • Easy to find someone to talk to about concerns • Family and friends given enough information to help recovery • Told about danger signals to watch for at home Also: percentage of smokers who quit and don't relapse

*VBAC indicates vaginal birth after cesarean delivery.

provide tools, techniques, and quality improvement expertise to the team. The project leader, however, drives the project on a daily basis (18).

Effective teams should be cross-functional and should include members with three types of expertise:

1. System leadership: someone with enough authority in the organization to institute change when it is suggested

2. Technical expertise: someone who understands the process of care being improved

3. Day-to-day leadership: someone who works on a daily basis in the process being improved (19).

To reduce redundancy, which occurs frequently in team meetings, it is suggested that team meetings not exceed 90 minutes and be held no more than weekly.

Data Collection and Information Sharing

Data collection is important not only in formulating the problem statement, but also to support the team's belief that a planned change will result in improvement. As mentioned previously in "Quality Improvement Projects," initial data collection is key for problem identification. Data also are critical for demonstrating that changes will result in system improvement. This is particularly helpful because not all change results in improvement.

It may not be necessary to collect volumes of data before effecting change. For example, sampling can be used to demonstrate the change being tested. Another suggestion is to use both qualitative and quantitative data. Process and outcome measures also may be used to help determine whether a change has led to improvement (19).

System Improvement

When the data gathered indicate that change will lead to improvement, the changes then can be implemented in a system-wide manner. Educational processes can be instituted in one or more of the following ways.

Clinical Protocols

Experts suggest that substantial quality improvements can be achieved by eliminating unnecessary variation in treatment plans (20). The QI committee can develop a draft protocol addressing a particular issue with the entire staff amending it to meet their needs. Once the protocol has been finalized, staff should be reminded that they may deviate from the protocol as long as the record reflects awareness of the protocol and documents the rationale and reasoning for not following it.

Department Meetings

Regular departmental meetings can be used to educate practitioners about improvement of quality of care. This might be a good forum to discuss documentation errors, including, for example, failure to include a treatment plan and to sign and date all notes in the record, as well as to discuss how to make a correction in the record. Regular meetings of the department also can be used to address specific clinical issues. This would allow the team member to present a problem case anonymously, discuss the issues, and review the literature and the methods that have been used by others to resolve the problem. Discussion can center around which practice guidelines can be incorporated into the department protocol and how to implement those changes. This method of teaching reinforces the need to improve processes at a department level rather than address the problem on an individual basis.

Presentations also may review complicated cases or difficult situations that were handled appropriately. These cases serve to identify which methods and treatments work well and can be used as the basis for protocols and improvement of care.

For small hospitals where effective peer review may be difficult because of antitrust or restraint of trade considerations, it may be helpful to develop a relationship with another hospital to conduct review. In other instances, it may be advisable to arrange for outside, independent peer review. In either case, it is important to remember that responsibility for peer review and quality improvement rests with the hospital medical staff and, ultimately, the governing board.

Grand Rounds or Other Continuing Education Programs

Variances identified through the ongoing QI process can be used to determine topics for continuing education programs. These programs may address topics such as laparoscopic complications and shoulder dystocia.

Summary of Morbidity Statistics

Periodically, the QI committee can present statistics for the department and share this with the staff to show them how they, as a department and individually, are doing. This would allow staff to understand the importance of what they are doing and how the changes they have instituted have had an impact on the quality of care.

Staff Letters

This method can be used to keep staff informed about changes and new protocols. Reminders about standards of care, trends in the department, and the need for documentation can be included regularly.

Electronic Transmission of Information

Many institutions and practitioners have access to electronic mail and fax machines. These methods of communication can be used to reinforce education and teaching. They also allow new information to be disseminated quickly and efficiently. The staff can be informed rapidly about a newly identified problem, recall of drugs, and defective instruments.

Corrective Action

When data analysis reveals an area of concern, a specific problem, or an opportunity to improve care or performance, a plan should be formulated to address the situation. It is important to first check applicable hospital and medical staff bylaws provisions to ensure that they will be followed. When deficiencies in care are found, the department chair, or the person designated by the medical staff bylaws, should investigate and take appropriate action. Such action may be department wide or directed toward one or more individuals. In the latter circumstance, the hospital's legal counsel should be consulted and involved in the process at an early stage to ensure compliance with the bylaws and due process. Corrective action usually can be handled within the department. However, specific problems that may require further investigation and corrective action should be handled as specified in the medical staff bylaws.

Performance profiles should be maintained by the QI committee. Once a practitioner's performance profile indicates that the standards of the department have not been met, corrective action may need to be instituted and documented. The severity of the problems will dictate the steps that need to be taken.

Opportunity for Improvement

At this level, the QI committee may meet with the practitioner to review concerns. The appropriate information to correct a perceived deficiency should be made available. The practitioner should be given educational materials concerning the particular problem that was identified. These materials may consist of protocols, current literature, or other related materials. Continued surveillance through record review may be all that is needed.

Deficiency of Care

If the QI committee concludes that a medical record reflects care that is inappropriate or of unacceptable quality, the problem should be referred to the appropriate body and documented as specified in the medical staff bylaws. Applicable confidentiality provisions must be followed. A member of the QI committee should be present at any hospital executive committee meeting at which the case is reviewed, to discuss the case and the reasons the care was deemed to be deficient.

Despite the best quality improvement efforts conducted by the department, there may be occasions when a physician outlier is identified whose quality of care is deficient and who is not willing or able to improve. These types of cases may require progressively severe steps of corrective action. There also may be cases where remedial steps have failed or have been refused, or where there is a pattern of inappropriate or substandard care, necessitating more severe disciplinary action.

The executive committee, the chair of the department, and the QI committee should determine which corrective steps should be taken. It should be emphasized that education is usually the initial response to most deviations from the standard of care, whether the deviation occurs within the activity of the department as a whole or within the practice of an individual physician. The following options should be considered:

- Meeting with the individual to discuss the care rendered
- Individual counseling
- Remedial and focused education
- Surveillance of care
- External peer review
- Supervision of care
- Probation within the department

- Restriction of privileges
- Dismissal from the department

Any recommendation that modifies a practitioner's privileges should be done in consultation with legal counsel and the hospital's governing board. The physician's confidential credentials file should document any discussion of the event that occurred, including the date, the individuals present, and the agreed-upon resolution. Final action on the department chair's recommendations for restriction of privileges is the ultimate responsibility of the hospital's governing board. Medical staff bylaws regarding due process should be followed during all stages of corrective actions. In addition, one must be aware of the reporting requirements of state medical boards and the federal National Practitioner Data Bank.

Ongoing review should occur to reassess the individual's quality of care. Once deficiencies have been corrected, removal of restrictions should be considered.

THE IMPAIRED OR DISRUPTIVE PHYSICIAN

Physician Impairment

The impaired physician presents a particularly sensitive problem to those engaged in peer review. Impairments are conditions or diseases that impede a physician's ability to practice, such as mental illness, alcoholism, chemical dependency, physical illness, or aging. Hospitals must have mechanisms in place to handle issues of impairment (21).

Identification

Early recognition of chemical dependency or other impairment can be difficult because of denial by a physician to family and peers. Such denial is common. Failure to follow patients appropriately, deterioration in the quality of medical records, frequent absences, and increased isolation from other staff members are common symptoms. Physicians' inappropriate prescriptions of excessive amounts of narcotics for themselves or family members are another indication.

Intervention

Too often, colleagues avoid dealing directly with a substance-abusing physician. However, physicians have a responsibility to recognize, assess, and report impairment. Failure to take action can result in serious consequences for patients, the hospital, and the physician, as evident in the following example.

EXAMPLE

A physician was noted to be increasingly erratic and disturbed. The physician's colleagues and the hospital administration suspected the impairment was the result of substance abuse. Rather than confront the problem, the administration counseled the physician and allowed him to move to another institution. In response to routine inquiries concerning his competence, both the medical staff and the administration failed to note their suspicions that a substance-abuse problem was present. When a serious injury occurred to a patient of this physician at the second institution, a lawsuit was filed, and the original hospital and medical staff were named as codefendants.

Intervention as soon as impairment is suspected or before professional performance is impaired should be encouraged. If intervention is to succeed, the following steps are important:

1. Obtain specific, well-documented evidence.

2. Consider using a group approach for the intervention. This group should include respected peers, a representative of the county or state medical society's impaired physician program, and a family member, if possible.

3. Use a nonjudgmental approach. This is vital if the physician's denial mechanism is to be broken.

4. Address the following questions:
   - Is there evidence of impaired ability to practice?
   - Is there imminent danger to patients?
   - Is there a history of previous treatment?
   - Is the physician motivated to enter a treatment program?

Treatment

Successful treatment plans, either inpatient or outpatient, must address both the type and severity of problems facing the impaired physician. Whenever possible, the personal preferences of the impaired physician should be taken into account.

Legal requirements applicable to the impaired physician vary from state to state. Some states investigate allegations of impairment, with the possibility of taking disciplinary action against the physician. Many require that impaired physicians' names be reported to the state medical board, whereas other states give confidentiality protection to physicians who voluntarily participate in treatment programs.

State medical societies with impaired physician programs currently represent the best source of information regarding the evaluation and treatment of impaired physicians and applicable legal requirements. These programs work with county medical societies, hospitals, and other self-help groups. Referrals may come from family, colleagues, hospital administrators, nurses, and other health care workers. These programs also provide follow-up and monitoring programs for impaired physicians.

The Disruptive Physician

Obstetrics and gynecology departments and physician practices should develop a policy for dealing with disruptive physicians whose behavior might include, among others, sexual harassment or temper tantrums. Suggestions include the following:

- Incorporate a written description of expected professional behavior into the group's or hospital's principles of practice and spell out the mechanisms for dealing with an emotionally disturbed, unruly, or generally disturbing individual.

- Establish a procedure for dealing with complaints and grievances from patients, peers, and staff, and identify communication consultants who offer skills training or counseling for troubled physicians.

- Provide each physician with regular feedback on his or her interpersonal skills and assist those who need to change their behavior.

- Insist that administrators be trained in confrontation skills so that they act before a disruptive physician emotionally damages the practice or hospital. Training can be provided by state medical societies' physician-assistance programs, individual consultants, or the staff of facilities for treatment of chemical or alcohol addiction (22).

COMPLIANCE

In addition to the accreditation and licensure survey programs that each facility, whether a hospital or outpatient clinic, must go through, two Joint Commission programs currently exist that are noteworthy.

Joint Commission Performance Measures Program

ORYX is the name of the Joint Commission's initiative to integrate outcomes and other performance measures into the accreditation process. Launched in 1997, the long-range goal of ORYX is to establish a data-driven, continuous survey and accreditation process to complement its standards-based assessment. Under the ORYX program, each accredited hospital is required to:

- Enroll in at least one performance measurement system chosen from those approved by the Joint Commission
- Identify six clinical measures to collect and submit to the designated system
- Inform the Joint Commission of the systems chosen and the measures selected

The hospital will then be required to submit data to the systems selected, which will in turn submit data reports to the Joint Commission. The systems will submit the individual organization's data for a given measure, along with comparative data on the performance of other organizations using the same measure.

Sentinel Event Policy

According to the Joint Commission, a "sentinel event is an unexpected occurrence involving death or serious physical or psychological injury, or the risk thereof." A serious injury specifically includes loss of limb or function, and the phrase "or the risk thereof" includes any process variation for which a recurrence would carry a significant chance of a serious adverse outcome.

The Joint Commission's Sentinel Event Policy is designed to encourage the self-reporting of medical errors to learn about the frequency and underlying causes of sentinel events, to share "lessons learned," and to reduce the risk of future sentinel events.

Under this policy, a defined set of sentinel events is reportable to the Joint Commission on a voluntary basis. The subset of sentinel events that is subject to review by the Joint Commission includes any occurrence that meets any of the following criteria:

- The event has resulted in an unanticipated death or major permanent loss of function, not related to the natural course of the patient's illness or underlying condition, or
- The event is one of the following (even if the outcome was not death or major permanent loss of function):
  - Suicide of a patient in a setting where the patient receives around-the-clock care
  - Infant abduction or discharge to the wrong family
  - Rape
  - Hemolytic transfusion reaction involving administration of blood or blood products having major blood group incompatibilities
  - Surgery on the wrong patient or wrong body part

Other examples of voluntarily reportable sentinel events include:

- Any intrapartum (related to the birth process) maternal death
- Any perinatal death unrelated to a congenital malformation in an infant having a birth weight greater than 2,500 g (23)

Under the sentinel event policy, each organization is encouraged, but not required, to report to the Joint Commission any sentinel event meeting the above criteria. If the Joint Commission becomes aware of the sentinel event, the organization is expected to prepare a thorough root-cause analysis and action plan.

Root-cause analysis is a process for identifying the basic or causal factors that underlie variation in performance. A root-cause analysis focuses primarily on systems and processes, not individual performance. The product of the root-cause analysis is an action plan that identifies the strategies that the organization intends to implement to reduce the risk of similar events occurring in the future. The plan should address responsibility for implementation, oversight, pilot testing as appropriate, timelines, and strategies for measuring the effectiveness of the actions (24).

Performing a root-cause analysis and developing an action plan is worthwhile even if not submitted to the Joint Commission. However, should this information be submitted to the Joint Commission, every effort should be made to ensure confidentiality. Although the Joint Commission ensures confidentiality of legally protected sentinel event–related information, it is nonetheless recommended that each hospital seek legal consultation before submitting reports to the Joint Commission.

PART 2

ASSESSING CLINICAL COMPETENCE

OVERVIEW

Credentialing and granting privileges to members of its medical staff are among the most important responsibilities of any health care facility. A multifaceted process, credentialing involves verification of licensure, education and training, malpractice experience, malpractice insurance coverage, and board certification as required by the facility. It requires requesting reports from the National Practitioner Data Bank and other facilities where the applicant has or has had privileges.

The more difficult, yet critical, aspect of this process is determining which requested privileges will be granted. Privileging defines what procedures a credentialed practitioner is permitted to perform at the facility. *The granting of privileges is based on training, experience, and demonstrated current clinical competence.* Each staff member must be assessed at the time of initial application as well as every 2 years at the time of reappraisal. In addition to routine requests for privileges, a physician also may request privileges to perform a new technology. The process of assessing current clinical competence and granting privileges is a difficult, time-consuming, yet critically necessary activity.

The purpose of this section is to provide guidance for these responsibilities. Privileges usually are formatted by levels (eg, Levels I, II, and III obstetric privileges and Levels I, II, and III gynecologic privileges). As new technologies evolve, processes for granting privileges for them will need to be formulated. For a sample application for privileges, which outlines such areas as emergency situations, provisional period, and the performance of new procedures, see Figure 4. Hospitals using

these materials may adapt them to conform to the specific situations at their facility. This information is not intended to be all inclusive or exclusive. It is intended primarily for educational purposes.

GRANTING PRIVILEGES

The following list has been developed to aid in granting privileges to those providers within the facility to perform obstetric and gynecologic procedures. The granting of privileges at any level in obstetrics and gynecology is based on satisfaction of criteria for the specified procedures. Criteria for granting privileges must be applied consistently regardless of the applicant's specialty. As stated, the granting of clinical privileges must be based on training, experience, and demonstrated current clinical competence. The educational requirements assume the achievement of a basic doctor of medicine or doctor of osteopathy degree.

I. Obstetric Privileges

A. Level I (Basic) Obstetric Privileges

1. Privileges may include (25):

a. Management of labor

b. Pudendal and local block anesthesia

c. Fetal assessment, antepartum and intrapartum, including limited obstetric ultrasound examination

d. Induction of labor

e. Internal fetal monitoring

This example is provided for educational purposes only. It may require modification for use in a particular facility.

1. Name _____

2. Department to which I am applying: _____

3. Other department(s) in which clinical privileges are held or sought: _____

_____

_____

4. Subject to consultation requirements and other policies, I understand that in exercising my clinical privileges granted, I am constrained by relevant Medical Center and Medical Policies requiring consultations for difficult diagnoses, conditions of extreme severity, and procedures and conditions that are beyond my area of training, specialization, and current competence and experience; by Medical Center policies concerning types of patients for whom it does not have appropriate resources (facilities, equipment, or personnel) to treat except on an emergency basis; and by such special policies as may from time to time be adopted.

5. Emergency situations:

   I also understand:

   (a) That the privileges are being requested for regular use in my practice

   (b) That it is not necessary to request "emergency" clinical privileges

   (c) That an emergency is deemed to exist whenever serious permanent harm or aggravation of injury or disease is imminent, or the life of a patient is in immediate danger, and any delay in administering treatment could add danger

   (d) That in such emergency, when better alternative sources of care are not reasonably available given the patient's condition, I am authorized and will be assisted to do everything possible to save the patient's life or to save the patient from serious harm to the degree permitted by my license but regardless of department affiliation or privileges

   (e) That if I provide services to a patient in an emergency, I am obligated to use appropriate consultative assistance when available and to arrange, when it is my responsibility, for appropriate follow-up care.

General Provisions

Basis for Granting Privileges

1. Applicants requesting clinical privileges must demonstrate satisfactory training, experience, and current competence for the privileges being requested and must agree to comply with the provisions contained in the medical staff bylaws.

2. Each applicant requesting privileges in the department of obstetrics and gynecology should be required to present his or her application and a list of recent cases for review by the department chief. (For physicians who have recently completed an ob-gyn program, the list could be the senior resident case list or the case

Fig. 4. Sample Application for Privileges: Department of Obstetrics and Gynecology

list submitted in conjunction with Part II of the board certification examination.) When family physicians or nurse midwives request privileges, an equivalent list of recently managed cases, representing the full range of privileges being requested, must also be submitted.

Provisional Period

1. All new appointees to the department of obstetrics and gynecology must undergo a minimum provisional period of no less than 12 months. The practitioner should have admitted a minimum number of cases to the hospital and/or completed an equivalent number of surgical procedures, as defined by the institution.

2. At his or her discretion, the chair may request any additional documentation deemed necessary to assess an applicant's competency in specific procedures during the provisional period.

   This documentation may include evidence of specific education or training in a procedure either during residency training or through postresidency courses.

3. At the conclusion of their provisional period, those individuals who did not meet the minimum criteria stipulated under Number 1 above or those who requested other than active staff status should provide the chair with a detailed listing of each case completed within the department as well as the description, scope, and breadth of their practice at other institutions. In addition to the hospital's QI review, the department chair also may request information from other institutions where the individual practices to assess overall competency for the procedure(s) requested.

4. Those individuals requesting privileges for a new procedure must have successfully completed their initial provisional period and have been appointed to the medical staff without restriction.

   They also should submit evidence they have completed an educational or training program in the specific procedure either in a residency program or through postgraduate residency training. In addition, each applicant should submit a letter from the director of a residency program stating that he or she is competent in the respective procedure and has completed the appropriate training.

   Individuals requesting privileges for a new procedure must be deemed competent to perform the procedure by an individual currently credentialed for that procedure in the department. However, if this is the first time these privileges have been requested within the department, arrangements should be made to ensure that the applicant is adequately evaluated before granting full, unrestricted privileges. In general, a minimum number of cases with preceptorship or observation, as defined by the institution, are required before full, unrestricted privileges can be granted for a new procedure.

New, Untried, Unproved, or Experimental Procedures and Treatment Modalities and Instrumentation

Experimental drugs, procedures, or other therapies or tests may be administered or performed only after approval of protocols involved by the committee responsible for the institutional review board function. Any other new, untried, or unproved procedure or treatment modality or instrumentation may be performed or used only after the regular credentialing process has been completed, and the privilege to perform or use said procedure or treatment modality or instrument has been granted to an individual practitioner. For the purposes of this paragraph, a new, untried, or unproved procedure or treatment modality or instrumentation is one that is *not* generalizable from an established procedure or treatment modality or instrumentation involving the same or similar skills, the same or similar instrumentation and technique, the same or similar complications, or same or similar indications as the established procedure or treatment modality or instrumentation.

Fig. 4. Sample Application for Privileges: Department of Obstetrics and Gynecology *(continued)*

f. Normal cephalic delivery, including use of vacuum extraction and outlet forceps

g. Episiotomy and repair, including third-degree lacerations

h. Management of common intrapartum problems

i. Exploration of vagina, cervix, and uterus

j. Emergency breech delivery

k. Management of common postpartum problems

l. First-assist at cesarean delivery

2. Training should include:

a. Obstetrician–gynecologist—successful completion of an Accreditation Council for Graduate Medical Education (ACGME)-accredited residency program in obstetrics and gynecology

b. Family physician—successful completion of a family practice residency that includes a curriculum of a minimum of 3 months in a structured obstetrics and gynecology rotation with substantial additional obstetric and gynecologic experience throughout the 3 years of their experience in family practice centers and in their continuity practices

3. Certification should be required:

a. Board certification (or active candidate) by the American Board of Obstetrics and Gynecology or the American Osteopathic Board of Obstetrics and Gynecology

b. Board certification (or active candidate) by the American Board of Family Physicians

c. Board recertification, if applicable

4. Reappraisal (recredentialing/reprivileging) (2-year cycle) should require:

a. Review of QI file:

(1) Trending

(2) Sentinel events

(3) Other problems with specific procedures

b. Review of level of activity:

(1) Total number of cases

(2) Total number of complications

(3) Outcomes

c. If the credentials committee determines that the number of cases performed within the cycle is insufficient for adequately assessing competency, it may recommend that the individual be proctored and evaluated for a designated period until competency is demonstrated. However, if the physician has privileges at another institution for the particular procedure, then the individual must provide credentialing data from that hospital for review by the credentials committee and may not require proctoring.

B. Level I (Advanced) Obstetric Privileges

1. Obtain additional intensified experience taught by or in collaboration with obstetrician–gynecologists (26). In programs where obstetrician–gynecologists are not available, these skills should be taught by appropriately skilled family physicians.

2. The assignment of hospital privileges is a local responsibility, and privileges should be granted on the basis of training, experience, and demonstrated current competence. All physicians should be held to the same standards for granting privileges, regardless of specialty, in order to assure the provision of high-quality patient care. Prearranged, collaborative relationships should be established to ensure ongoing consultations, as well as consultations needed for emergencies.

The standard of training should allow any physician who receives training in a cognitive or surgical skill to meet the criteria for privileges in that area of practice. Provisional privileges in primary care, obstetric care, and cesarean delivery should be granted regardless of specialty as long as training criteria and experience are documented. All physicians should be subject to a proctorship period to allow demonstration of ability and current competence. These principles should apply to all health care systems.

3. Privileges recommended by the department of family practice shall be the responsibility of the department of family practice. Similarly, privileges recommended by the

department of obstetrics and gynecology shall be the responsibility of the department of obstetrics and gynecology. When privileges are recommended jointly by the departments of family practice and obstetrics and gynecology, they shall be the joint responsibility of the two departments.

C. Level II (Specialty) Obstetric Privileges

    1. Privileges may include:

        a. All Level I obstetric privileges

        b. Management of normal and abnormal labor and delivery (including premature labor, breech presentation, cesarean delivery, vaginal delivery after previous cesarean delivery, cephalopelvic disproportion, nonreassuring fetal status, use of amniotomy and oxytocin, and midforceps delivery)

        c. Management of medical or surgical complications of pregnancy

        d. Diagnostic amniocentesis

        e. Cesarean hysterectomy

        f. Hypogastric artery ligation

        g. Repair of incompetent cervix

        h. External version of breech presentation

        i. Obstetric ultrasonography—complete

        j Midforceps rotation

        k. Regional anesthesia as determined by training and local practice

    2. Training requires successful completion of an ACGME-accredited residency program in obstetrics and gynecology

    3. Certification should be required:

        a. Board certification (or active candidate) by the American Board of Obstetrics and Gynecology in general obstetrics and gynecology or in maternal–fetal medicine

        b. Board recertification, if applicable

    4. Reappraisal (recredentialing/reprivileging) (2-year cycle) should require:

        a. Review of QI file:

            (1) Trending

            (2) Sentinel events

            (3) Other problems with specific procedures

        b. Review of level of activity:

            (1) Total number of cases

            (2) Total number of complications

            (3) Outcomes

        c. If the credentials committee determines that the number of cases performed within the cycle is insufficient for adequately assessing competency, it may recommend that the individual be proctored and evaluated for a designated period until competency is demonstrated. However, if the physician has privileges at another institution for the particular procedure, then the individual must provide credentialing data from that hospital for review by the credentials committee and may not require proctoring.

D. Level III (Subspecialty) Obstetric Privileges

    1. Privileges may include:

        a. All Level I and II obstetric privileges

        b. Intrauterine fetal transfusion

        c. Intrauterine fetal surgery

        d. Chorionic villous sampling

        e. Percutaneous umbilical sampling

    2. Training should include:

        a. Successful completion of an ACGME-accredited residency program in obstetrics and gynecology

        b. Documentation of specialized postresidency training

    3. Certification should be required:

        a. Board certification (or active candidate) by the American Board of Obstetrics and Gynecology in general obstetrics and gynecology or in maternal–fetal medicine

        b. Board recertification, if applicable

    4. Reappraisal (recredentialing/reprivileging) (2-year cycle) should require:

        a. Review of QI file:

            (1) Trending

            (2) Sentinel events

            (3) Other problems with specific procedures

b. Review of level of activity:

(1) Total number of cases

(2) Total number of complications

(3) Outcomes

c. If the credentials committee determines that the number of cases performed within the cycle is insufficient for adequately assessing competency, it may recommend that the individual be proctored and evaluated for a designated period until competency is demonstrated. However, if the physician has privileges at another institution for the particular procedure, then the individual must provide credentialing data from that hospital for review by the credentials committee and may not require proctoring.

II. Gynecologic Privileges

A. Level I (Basic) Gynecologic Privileges

1. Privileges may include (25):

a. Appropriate screening examination of the female, including breast examination

b. Obtaining vaginal and cervical cytology

c. Colposcopy

d. Cervical biopsy, polypectomy

e. Endometrial biopsy

f. Culdocentesis

g. Cryosurgery/cautery for benign disease

h. Microscopic diagnosis of urine and vaginal smears

i. Bartholin duct cyst drainage or marsupialization

j. Dilation and curettage for incomplete abortion

2. Training should include:

a. Obstetrician–gynecologist—successful completion of an ACGME-accredited residency program in obstetrics and gynecology

b. Family physician—successful completion of a family practice residency that includes a curriculum of a minimum of 3 months in a structured obstetrics and gynecology rotation with substantial additional obstetric and gynecologic experience

throughout the 3 years of experience in family practice centers and in their continuity practices

c. Documentation of appropriate training and experience for physicians performing Level I procedures

3. Certification should be required:

a. Board certification (or active candidate) by the American Board of Family Physicians *or*

b. Board certification (or active candidate) by the American Board of Obstetrics and Gynecology

c. Board recertification, if applicable

4. Reappraisal (recredentialing/reprivileging) (2-year cycle) should require:

a. Review of QI file:

(1) Trending

(2) Sentinel events

(3) Other problems with specific procedures

b. Review of level of activity:

(1) Total number of cases

(2) Total number of complications

(3) Outcomes

c. If the credentials committee determines that the number of cases performed within the cycle is insufficient for adequately assessing competency, it may recommend that the individual be proctored and evaluated for a designated period until competency is demonstrated. However, if the physician has privileges at another institution for the particular procedure, then the individual must provide credentialing data from that hospital for review by the credentials committee and may not require proctoring.

B. Level II (Specialty) Gynecologic Privileges

1. Privileges may include:

a. All Level I gynecologic privileges

b. Dilation and curettage, with or without biopsy

c. Dilation and curettage, with or without conization

d. Laparotomy

e. Operations for removal of uterus, cervix, oviducts, ovaries (abdominal or vaginal), and appendix

f. Diagnostic laparoscopy

g. Tubal sterilization

h. Operations for treatment of urinary stress incontinence, vaginal approach, retropubic urethral suspension, or sling procedure

i. Fistula repairs (vesicovaginal or rectovaginal)

j. Tuboplasty (micro, macro, fimbrioplasty)

k. Hernia repair (incisional or umbilical)

l. Operations for treatment of noninvasive carcinoma of vulva, vagina, uterus, ovary, and cervix

m. Repair of rectocele, enterocele

n. Vaginectomy (total or partial)

o. Colpocleisis

p. Strassman procedure (metroplasty)

q. Myomectomy

r. Node dissection (superficial inguinal, pelvic, or paraaortic)

s. Diagnostic hysteroscopy

t. Second-trimester abortion by medical or surgical means

2. Training should include successful completion of an ACGME-accredited residency program in obstetrics and gynecology

3. Certification should be required:

a. Board certification (or active candidate) by the American Board of Obstetrics and Gynecology

b. Board recertification, if applicable

4. Reappraisal (recredentialing/reprivileging) (2-year cycle) should require:

a. Review of QI file:

(1) Trending

(2) Sentinel events

(3) Other problems with specific procedures

b. Review of level of activity:

(1) Total number of cases

(2) Total number of complications

(3) Outcomes

c. If the credentials committee determines that the number of cases performed within the cycle is insufficient for adequately assessing competency, it may recommend that the individual be proctored and evaluated for a designated period until competency is demonstrated. However, if the physician has privileges at another institution for the particular procedure, then the individual must provide credentialing data from that hospital for review by the credentials committee and may not require proctoring.

C. Level III-A: Basic Endoscopic Procedures

1. Privileges may include:

a. All Level I and II gynecologic privileges

b. Endoscopic ovarian or endometrial biopsy

c. Needle aspiration of simple cysts

d. Minor adhesiolysis

e. Management of ectopic pregnancy (linear salpingostomy, partial salpingectomy)

f. Destruction of endometriosis stage I and stage II as graded by American Society of Reproductive Medicine criteria

2. Training should include successful completion of an ACGME-accredited residency program in obstetrics and gynecology

3. Certification should be required:

a. Board certification (or active candidate) by The American Board of Obstetrics and Gynecology

b. Board recertification, if applicable

4. Experience should be required:

a. The applicant must possess the proficiency and be privileged to perform the requested procedures in an open (laparotomy) manner

b. The applicant should have been granted privileges to perform basic (Level III-A) endoscopic procedures and should have demonstrated competency in these techniques

5. Reappraisal (recredentialing/reprivileging) (2-year cycle) should require:

a. Review of QI file:

(1) Trending

(2) Sentinel events

(3) Other problems with specific procedures

b. Review of level of activity

(1) Total number of cases

(2) Total number of complications

(3) Outcomes

c. If the credentials committee determines that the number of cases performed within the cycle is insufficient for adequately assessing competency, it may recommend that the individual be proctored and evaluated for a designated period until competency is demonstrated. However, if the physician has privileges at another institution for the particular procedure, then the individual must provide credentialing data from that hospital for review by the credentials committee and may not require proctoring.

D. Level III-B: Advanced Endoscopic Procedures

1. Privileges may include:

a. All Level I and II gynecologic privileges

b. Laparoscopically assisted vaginal hysterectomy

c. Laparoscopic ovarian cystectomy

d. Salpingo-oophorectomy

e. Adhesiolysis

f. Management of endometriosis, stage III and IV

g. Division of the uterosacral ligaments

h. Appendectomy

i. Operative hysteroscopy requiring use of the resectoscope (division or resection of the uterine septum, surgical treatment of Asherman's syndrome, resection of uterine myomas)

j. Myomectomy

k. Pelvic lymphadenectomy

l. Pelvic sidewall dissection

m. Ureteral dissection

n. Presacral neurectomy

o. Dissection of obliterated pouch of Douglas

p. Hernia repair

q. Retropubic bladder neck suspension

r. Sling procedure

s. Bowel surgery

2. Training should require:

a. Successful completion of an ACGME-accredited residency program in obstetrics and gynecology, *and*

b. Successful completion of advanced training that includes training in listed procedures, or documented course, including didactic and hands-on laboratory experience, unless included in residency program

3. Certification should be required:

a. Board certification (or active candidate) by the American Board of Obstetrics and Gynecology

b. Board recertification, if applicable

4. Experience should include advanced procedures requiring the following additional training and documentation:

a. Completion of a postgraduate course, accredited by the Accreditation Council for Continuing Medical Education (ACCME), that includes didactic training (must include education on equipment operation and safety factors) and hands-on laboratory experience, *and*

b. Preceptorship

If not included in residency training, the applicant must:

(1) Complete a preceptorship with a physician already credentialed to perform the procedures of that skill level; the preceptorship should require the applicant to perform the designated surgery with the preceptor acting as first assistant

(2) Provide a list of cases satisfactorily completed under supervision at each skill level, as defined by the local institution

(3) Submit a letter from the preceptor documenting that the procedures were completed in a satisfactory manner and that the applicant is competent to perform the procedures independently at the designated skill level.

If there is no experienced surgeon on the hospital staff who is able to serve as a preceptor for advanced or new surgical procedures, a supervised preceptorship must be arranged. This may be done by scheduling a number of cases from physicians requiring credentialing and inviting a credentialed surgeon from another institution to serve as a surgical consultant.

   c. In the event that credentials in advanced endoscopy are already established at a different hospital, the applicant must present evidence of these established credentials in lieu of (a) and (b) above. In addition, the applicant must provide a list of cases performed over the past 24 months, including preoperative and postoperative diagnoses, procedure, type of endoscope used, outcome, and complications of the procedure.

   d. A letter from the director of an approved residency program can substitute for (a) and (b) above. In addition, this new residency graduate must provide a list of advanced endoscopy cases performed over the past 24 months.

5. Reappraisal (recredentialing/reprivileging) (2-year cycle) should require:

   a. Review of QI file:

     (1) Trending

     (2) Sentinel events

     (3) Other problems with specific procedures

   b. Review of level of activity:

     (1) Total number of cases

     (2) Total number of complications

     (3) Outcomes

   c. If the credentials committee determines that the number of cases performed within the cycle is insufficient for adequately assessing competency, it may recommend that the individual be proctored and evaluated for a designated period until competency is demonstrated. However, if the physician has privileges at another institution for the particular procedure, then the individual must provide credentialing data from that hospital for review by the credentials committee and may not require proctoring.

E. Level III-C: Gynecologic Oncology

1. Privileges (in addition to Level I and Level II procedures) may include:

   a. Treatment of malignant disease with chemotherapy

   b. Radical hysterectomy for treatment of invasive carcinoma of the cervix

   c. Radical surgery for treatment of gynecologic malignancy to include procedures on bowel, ureter, or bladder, as indicated

   d. Treatment of invasive carcinoma of vulva by radical vulvectomy

   e. Treatment of invasive carcinoma of the vagina by radical vaginectomy and other appropriate surgery

2. Training should include:

   a. Successful completion of an ACGME-accredited residency program in obstetrics and gynecology

   b. Documentation of specialized postresidency training or experience or both

3. Certification should be required:

   a. Board certification (or active candidate) by the American Board of Obstetrics and Gynecology in general obstetrics and gynecology or in gynecologic oncology

   b. Board recertification, if applicable

4. Reappraisal (recredentialing/reprivileging) (2-year cycle) should require:

   a. Review of QI file:

     (1) Trending

     (2) Sentinel events

     (3) Other problems with specific procedures

   b. Review of level of activity:

     (1) Total number of cases

     (2) Total number of complications

     (3) Outcomes

   c. If the credentials committee determines that the number of cases performed within the cycle is insufficient for adequately assessing competency, it may recommend that the individual be proctored and evaluated for a designated period until competency is demonstrated. However, if the physician has privileges at another institution for the particular procedure, then the individual must provide credentialing data from that hospital for review by the credentials committee and may not require proctoring.

d. If there is no experienced surgeon on the hospital staff who is able to serve as a preceptor for advanced or new surgical procedures, a supervised preceptorship must be arranged. This may be done by scheduling a number of cases from physicians requiring credentialing and inviting a credentialed surgeon from another institution to serve as a surgical consultant.

F. Level III-D: Assisted Reproductive Techniques

1. Privileges may include:

   a. Gynecologic Levels I, II, III-A, and III-B

   b. In vitro fertilization and gamete intrafallopian transfer

2. Training should include:

   a. Successful completion of an ACGME-accredited residency program in obstetrics and gynecology *and*

   b. Documentation of training and experience in reproductive endocrinology and pelvic reproductive surgery, including experience in operative laparoscopic procedures *and*

   c. Documentation of training and experience in in vitro fertilization–embryo transfer and gamete intrafallopian transfer procedures

3. Certification should be required:

   a. Board certification (or active candidate) by the American Board of Obstetrics and Gynecology in general obstetrics and gynecology or in reproductive endocrinology and infertility

   b. Board recertification, if applicable

4. Experience should require demonstrating knowledge of all aspects of assisted reproductive techniques

5. Reappraisal (recredentialing/reprivileging) (2-year cycle) should require:

   a. Review of QI file:

      (1) Trending

      (2) Sentinel events

      (3) Other problems with specific procedures

   b. Review of level of activity:

      (1) Total number of cases

      (2) Total number of complications

      (3) Outcomes

   c. If the credentials committee determines that the number of cases performed within the cycle is insufficient for adequately assessing competency, it may recommend that the individual be proctored and evaluated for a designated period until competency is demonstrated. However, if the physician has privileges at another institution for the particular procedure, then the individual must provide credentialing data from that hospital for review by the credentials committee and may not require proctoring.

   d. If there is no experienced surgeon on the hospital staff who is able to serve as a preceptor for advanced or new surgical procedures, a supervised preceptorship must be arranged. This may be done by scheduling a number of cases from physicians requiring credentialing and inviting a credentialed surgeon from another institution to serve as a surgical consultant.

G. Level III-E: Laser Therapy

1. Privileges may include:

   a. Laser therapy for cervix, vagina, vulva, and perineum (colposcopically directed)

   b. Conization of cervix

   c. Lysis of adhesions and photocoagulation (intraabdominal "free hand use")

   d. Lysis of adhesions and photocoagulation (microscopically directed)

   e. Oncologic debulking procedures (intraabdominal "free hand use")

2. Training should include:

   a. Successful completion of an ACGME-accredited residency program in obstetrics and gynecology *and*

   b. Documentation of laser training from a residency program director, attesting to the completion of at least 8 hours observation and hands-on involvement, *or*

   c. Documentation of a laser training course, including laser physics, safety, indications and complications, and hands-on experience

3. Certification should be required:

   a. Board certification (or active candidate) by the American Board of Obstetrics and Gynecology

   b. Board recertification, if applicable

4. Experience should include:

   a. Level II gynecologic privileges *and*

   b. Laser privileges as defined on the hospital-wide laser privilege request form

5. Reappraisal (recredentialing/reprivileging) (2-year cycle) should require:

   a. Review of QI file:

      (1) Trending

      (2) Sentinel events

      (3) Other problems with specific procedures

   b. Review of level of activity:

      (1) Total number of cases

      (2) Total number of complications

      (3) Outcomes

   c. If the credentials committee determines that the number of cases performed within the cycle is insufficient for adequately assessing competency, it may recommend that the individual be proctored and evaluated for a designated period until competency is demonstrated. However, if the physician has privileges at another institution for the particular procedure, then the individual must provide credentialing data from that hospital for review by the credentials committee and may not require proctoring.

   d. If there is no experienced surgeon on the hospital staff who is able to serve as a preceptor for advanced or new surgical procedures, a supervised preceptorship must be arranged. This may be done by scheduling a number of cases from physicians requiring credentialing and inviting a credentialed surgeon from another institution to serve as a surgical consultant.

H. Level III-F: Endometrial Ablation

   1. Privileges may include:

      a. Laser ablation

      b. Electrosurgical ablation

      c. Thermal balloon ablation

      d. Other techniques

   2. Training should include:

      a. Laser ablation

         (1) Successful completion of an ACGME-accredited residency program in obstetrics and gynecology *and*

         (2) Documentation from residency program director, attesting to the completion of least 8 hours of observation and hands-on involvement *or*

         (3) Documentation of an operative hysteroscopy and laser ablation of the endometrium course, including laser physics, safety, indications and complications, and hands-on experience

      b. Electrosurgical ablation

         (1) Successful completion of an ACGME-accredited residency program in obstetrics and gynecology *and*

         (2) Documentation from residency program director, including at least 8 hours of observation and hands-on involvement, *or*

         (3) Documentation of competency and demonstration of hands-on experience in operative hysteroscopy with endometrial rollerball

      c. Thermal balloon ablation

         (1) Successful completion of an ACGME-accredited residency program in obstetrics and gynecology *and*

(2) Documentation from residency program director, attesting to the completion of at least 8 hours of observation and hands-on involvement *or*

(3) Documentation of competency and demonstration of hands-on experience

3. Certification should be required:

a. Board certification (or active candidate) by the American Board of Obstetrics and Gynecology

b. Board recertification, if applicable

4. Experience should include proficiency in diagnostic hysteroscopy if laser or electrosurgical ablation is performed

5. Reappraisal (recredentialing/reprivileging) (2-year cycle) should require:

a. Review of QI file:

(1) Trending

(2) Sentinel events

(3) Other problems with specific procedures

b. Review of level of activity:

(1) Total number of cases

(2) Total number of complications

(3) Outcomes

c. If the credentials committee determines that the number of cases performed within the cycle is insufficient for adequately assessing competency, it may recommend that the individual be proctored and evaluated for a designated period until competency is demonstrated. However, if the physician has privileges at another institution for the particular procedure, then the individual must provide credentialing data from that hospital for review by the credentials committee and may not require proctoring.

d. If there is no experienced surgeon on the hospital staff who is able to serve as a preceptor for advanced or new surgical procedures, a supervised preceptorship must be arranged. This may be done by scheduling a number of cases from physicians requiring credentialing and inviting a credentialed surgeon from another institution to serve as a surgical consultant.

REQUESTS FOR NEW PRIVILEGES

New Equipment and Technology

New equipment or technology usually improves health care, provided that practitioners and other hospital staff understand the proper indications for usage. Problems can arise when staff perform duties or use equipment for which they are not trained. It is imperative that all staff be properly trained in the use of the advanced technology or new equipment.

One should consider granting privileges for new skills (eg, laparoscopic morcellator, harmonic scalpel) only when the appropriate training has been completed and documented and the competency level has been achieved with adequate supervision. That is, each physician requesting additional privileges for new equipment or technology should be evaluated by answering the following questions:

1. Does the hospital have a mechanism in place to ensure that necessary support for the new equipment or technology is available?

2. Has the physician been adequately trained, including hands-on experience, to use the new equipment or to perform the new technology?

3. Has the physician adequately demonstrated an ability to use the new equipment or perform the new technology? This may require that the physician undergo a period of proctoring or supervision, or both. If no one on staff can serve as a proctor, the hospital may either require reciprocal proctoring at another hospital or grant temporary privileges to someone from another hospital to supervise the applicant.

After a Period of Inactivity

There may be instances when a physician returns to practice after a period of inactivity or requests privileges for procedures that he or she has not practiced for several years (eg, obstetrics). In these cases, a general guideline for evaluation would be to consider the physician as any other new applicant for privileges. This would include evaluation of the following:

1. Demonstration that a minimum number of hours of continuing medical education has been earned during the period of inactivity

2. In accordance with the medical staff bylaws, supervision by a proctor appointed by the department chair for a minimum number of cases during the provisional period

3. Further review of cases as required by the departmental quality improvement committee.

PART 3

ACOG SCREENING TOOLS

The name *Criteria Sets* was used by ACOG to identify documents designed to be used by nonphysicians with some medical record training (eg, a health record analyst) as a first screen to identify charts that may or may not comply with the current standard of care. The name was often misconstrued to imply that these documents could be used to determine whether a case complied with medical standards. Because this was not the intended purpose for these documents, a new name, ACOG Screening Tool, was selected to describe their intended function more adequately. If a medical record is flagged by this first screen, the record should then be reviewed by a qualified physician to determine the appropriateness of the issues in question. This initial screen is not designed to determine if charts are not in compliance with the medical standards. Only the qualified physician reviewer can determine the appropriateness of care. A sample medical record review methodology can be found in Figure 5.

The Criteria Sets also were not designed to determine appropriateness for reimbursement. It is intended that the new name also will deter this misapplication of the documents.

Current procedural terminology (CPT) five-digit codes, nomenclature, and other data are copyright 1999 American Medical Association. All rights reserved. No fee schedules, basic units, relative values, or related listings are included in CPT. The AMA assumes no liability for the data contained herein.

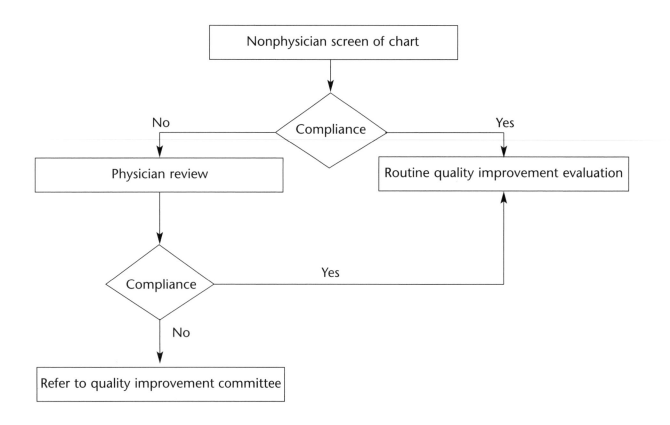

Fig. 5. Sample Medical Record Review Methods

ACOG Screening Tool

Cesarean Delivery for Failure to Progress

STATEMENT REGARDING THE USE OF SCREENING TOOLS. The American College of Obstetricians and Gynecologists (ACOG), through the Committee on Quality Assessment, develops Screening Tools to assist in retrospective chart review to evaluate quality of patient care. They are based primarily on ACOG publications and consensus opinions and do not necessarily mention all acceptable clinical approaches. Departments of obstetrics and gynecology may modify these criteria to reflect local practice. The purpose of Screening Tools is to aid in identifying practice variances that might indicate the need for further review, documentation, or justification. Only peer review can determine whether such variations are appropriate. The use of Screening Tools alone for utilization review or as the basis to deny reimbursement for health services is inappropriate.

It is important to understand that Screening Tools are particularly useful in screening cases of morbidity and mortality. However, Screening Tools that address procedures or diagnoses lack specificity or sensitivity, or both; consequently, their usefulness is limited. In using Screening Tools that address procedures or diagnoses, many charts fail the screen, but relatively few, after physician review, are determined to represent quality issues.

Purpose

The purpose of this Screening Tool is to identify cases that may require physician review because they fail to meet the listed criteria for screening patients undergoing cesarean delivery for the indication of failure to progress. Identified cases may require physician review for QI purposes.

Procedure

Cesarean delivery (ICD-9-CM Procedural Codes 74.0 or 74.1 (**CPT* Codes 59510** or **59618** [global service], **59514** or **59620** [delivery only], or **59515** or **59622** [delivery and postpartum care only])

Indication

The major single indication for cesarean delivery is failure to progress (lack of progress). Reasons for lack of progress include disproportion (ICD 9-CM Code 653.XX); primary uterine inertia (661.0X); secondary uterine inertia (661.1X); other and unspecified uterine inertia (661.2X); prolonged first stage (662.0X); prolonged labor, unspecified (662.1X); and prolonged second stage (662.2X).

---

*CPT only © 1999 American Medical Association. All rights reserved.

Screening Criteria

Cesarean Delivery for Failure to Progress

Unless otherwise indicated, any time an unshaded box is checked, the chart should be referred for physician review.

Were the following documented in the medical record?	Yes	No
1. Absence of cervical dilatation after at least 2 hours of active phase of labor or no descent of presenting part for at least 1 hour during the second stage of labor with the patient in active labor	■	☐
2. Active labor as defined by (a *and* b)		
a. Cervix dilated to at least 3 cm in nullipara or 4 cm in multipara	■	☐
b. Adequate frequency and intensity of uterine activity	■	☐
3. Ruptured membranes	■	☐
4. Oxytocin infusion for inadequate contractions when progressive cervical dilation or descent of presenting part fails to occur in the active phase of labor	■	☐
5. Anesthesia consultation and evaluation	■	☐
6. Fetal heart rate monitored before preparation of abdomen	■	☐
7. Qualified personnel* in attendance for resuscitation and care of newborn	■	☐
8. Vaginal examination before surgery to confirm failure to progress	■	☐

* As determined by the hospital

STATEMENT REGARDING THE USE OF SCREENING TOOLS. The American College of Obstetricians and Gynecologists (ACOG), through the Committee on Quality Assessment, develops Screening Tools to assist in retrospective chart review to evaluate quality of patient care. They are based primarily on ACOG publications and consensus opinions and do not necessarily mention all acceptable clinical approaches. Departments of obstetrics and gynecology may modify these criteria to reflect local practice. The purpose of Screening Tools is to aid in identifying practice variances that might indicate the need for further review, documentation, or justification. Only peer review can determine whether such variations are appropriate. The use of Screening Tools alone for utilization review or as the basis to deny reimbursement for health services is inappropriate. It is important to understand that Screening Tools are particularly useful in screening cases of morbidity and mortality. However, Screening Tools that address procedures or diagnoses lack specificity or sensitivity, or both; consequently, their usefulness is limited. In using Screening Tools that address procedures or diagnoses, many charts fail the screen, but relatively few, after physician review, are determined to represent quality issues.

ACOG SCREENING TOOL

___

CESAREAN DELIVERY FOR NONREASSURING FETAL STATUS

STATEMENT REGARDING THE USE OF SCREENING TOOLS. The American College of Obstetricians and Gynecologists (ACOG), through the Committee on Quality Assessment, develops Screening Tools to assist in retrospective chart review to evaluate quality of patient care. They are based primarily on ACOG publications and consensus opinions and do not necessarily mention all acceptable clinical approaches. Departments of obstetrics and gynecology may modify these criteria to reflect local practice. The purpose of Screening Tools is to aid in identifying practice variances that might indicate the need for further review, documentation, or justification. Only peer review can determine whether such variations are appropriate. The use of Screening Tools alone for utilization review or as the basis to deny reimbursement for health services is inappropriate.

It is important to understand that Screening Tools are particularly useful in screening cases of morbidity and mortality. However, Screening Tools that address procedures or diagnoses lack specificity or sensitivity, or both; consequently, their usefulness is limited. In using Screening Tools that address procedures or diagnoses, many charts fail the screen, but relatively few, after physician review, are determined to represent quality issues.

Purpose

The purpose of this Screening Tool is to identify those cases that may require physician review because they fail to meet the listed criteria for screening patients undergoing cesarean delivery for the indication of nonreassuring fetal status. Identified cases may require physician review for QI purposes.

Procedure

Cesarean delivery (ICD-9-CM Procedural Codes 74.0 or 74.1) (**CPT* Codes 59510 or 59618**)

Indication

Nonreassuring fetal status (ICD-9-CM Codes 656.83 or 659.73 if affecting management of mother antepartum; ICD-9-CM Codes 656.81 or 659.71 if affecting management of mother delivered)

Bibliography

American College of Obstetricians and Gynecologists. Fetal heart rate patterns: monitoring, interpretation, and management. ACOG Technical Bulletin 207. Washington, DC: ACOG, 1995

___

*CPT only © 1999 American Medical Association. All rights reserved.

Screening Criteria

Cesarean Delivery for Nonreassuring Fetal Status

Unless otherwise indicated, any time an unshaded box is checked, the chart should be referred for physician review.

Were the following documented in the medical record?   Yes   No

1. Patient history of (a *or* b *or* c)   ■   ❏
   a. Recurrent late, prolonged, or severe variable decelerations
   b. Sinusoidal pattern
   c. Prolonged bradycardia

2. Repositioning of patient   ■   ❏

3. Administration of oxygen to mother   ■   ❏

4. Discontinuation of uterine stimulants (eg, oxytocin) and attempt at correction of uterine
   hyperstimulation, if present   ■   ❏

5. Vaginal examination   ■   ❏

6. Maternal vital signs   ■   ❏

7. Correction of maternal hypotension associated with regional anesthesia, if present   ■   ❏

STATEMENT REGARDING THE USE OF SCREENING TOOLS. The American College of Obstetricians and Gynecologists (ACOG), through the Committee on Quality Assessment, develops Screening Tools to assist in retrospective chart review to evaluate quality of patient care. They are based primarily on ACOG publications and consensus opinions and do not necessarily mention all acceptable clinical approaches. Departments of obstetrics and gynecology may modify these criteria to reflect local practice. The purpose of Screening Tools is to aid in identifying practice variances that might indicate the need for further review, documentation, or justification. Only peer review can determine whether such variations are appropriate. The use of Screening Tools alone for utilization review or as the basis to deny reimbursement for health services is inappropriate. It is important to understand that Screening Tools are particularly useful in screening cases of morbidity and mortality. However, Screening Tools that address procedures or diagnoses lack specificity or sensitivity, or both; consequently, their usefulness is limited. In using Screening Tools that address procedures or diagnoses, many charts fail the screen, but relatively few, after physician review, are determined to represent quality issues.

ACOG SCREENING TOOL

EXTERNAL CEPHALIC VERSION

STATEMENT REGARDING THE USE OF SCREENING TOOLS. The American College of Obstetricians and Gynecologists (ACOG), through the Committee on Quality Assessment, develops Screening Tools to assist in retrospective chart review to evaluate quality of patient care. They are based primarily on ACOG publications and consensus opinions and do not necessarily mention all acceptable clinical approaches. Departments of obstetrics and gynecology may modify these criteria to reflect local practice. The purpose of Screening Tools is to aid in identifying practice variances that might indicate the need for further review, documentation, or justification. Only peer review can determine whether such variations are appropriate. The use of Screening Tools alone for utilization review or as the basis to deny reimbursement for health services is inappropriate.

It is important to understand that Screening Tools are particularly useful in screening cases of morbidity and mortality. However, Screening Tools that address procedures or diagnoses lack specificity or sensitivity, or both; consequently, their usefulness is limited. In using Screening Tools that address procedures or diagnoses, many charts fail the screen, but relatively few, after physician review, are determined to represent quality issues.

Purpose

The purpose of this Screening Tool is to identify those cases that may require physician review because they fail to meet criteria for screening patients undergoing antepartum external cephalic version. Identified cases may require physician review for QI purposes.

Procedure

Antepartum external cephalic version (ICD-9-CM Procedural Code 73.91) (**CPT* Code 59412 with or without 52 modifier**)

---

*CPT only © 1999 American Medical Association. All rights reserved.

Indications

Breech or transverse lie (ICD-9-CM Codes 652.13 and 652.23 or 652.33)

Bibliography

American College of Obstetricians and Gynecologists. Management of the breech presentation. ACOG Technical Bulletin 95. Washington, DC: ACOG, 1986

American College of Obstetricians and Gynecologists. External cephalic version. ACOG Practice Bulletin 13. Washington, DC: ACOG, 2000

Screening Criteria

External Cephalic Version

Unless otherwise indicated, any time an unshaded box is checked, the chart should be referred for physician review.

Were the following documented in the medical record?   Yes   No

1. Before the procedure:
   a. Normal fetal assessment study (eg, nonstress test or biophysical profile)   ■   ❑
   b. Rh status   ■   ❑
   c. Ultrasound assessment to confirm noncephalic presentation and to exclude placenta previa
      and lethal fetal anomalies   ■   ❑

2. During or following the procedure:
   a. Monitoring the fetal heart rate   ■   ❑
   b. Monitoring procedure with ultrasonography   ■   ❑
   c. Administering anti-D immune globulin if indicated   ■   ❑

3. Before discharge:
   a. Observation of patient for pain, bleeding, or labor   ■   ❑
   b. Confirmation of normal fetal heart rate   ■   ❑

STATEMENT REGARDING THE USE OF SCREENING TOOLS. The American College of Obstetricians and Gynecologists (ACOG), through the Committee on Quality Assessment, develops Screening Tools to assist in retrospective chart review to evaluate quality of patient care. They are based primarily on ACOG publications and consensus opinions and do not necessarily mention all acceptable clinical approaches. Departments of obstetrics and gynecology may modify these criteria to reflect local practice. The purpose of Screening Tools is to aid in identifying practice variances that might indicate the need for further review, documentation, or justification. Only peer review can determine whether such variations are appropriate. The use of Screening Tools alone for utilization review or as the basis to deny reimbursement for health services is inappropriate. It is important to understand that Screening Tools are particularly useful in screening cases of morbidity and mortality. However, Screening Tools that address procedures or diagnoses lack specificity or sensitivity, or both; consequently, their usefulness is limited. In using Screening Tools that address procedures or diagnoses, many charts fail the screen, but relatively few, after physician review, are determined to represent quality issues.

ACOG Screening Tool

Hospitalization for Preeclampsia

STATEMENT REGARDING THE USE OF SCREENING TOOLS. The American College of Obstetricians and Gynecologists (ACOG), through the Committee on Quality Assessment, develops Screening Tools to assist in retrospective chart review to evaluate quality of patient care. They are based primarily on ACOG publications and consensus opinions and do not necessarily mention all acceptable clinical approaches. Departments of obstetrics and gynecology may modify these criteria to reflect local practice. The purpose of Screening Tools is to aid in identifying practice variances that might indicate the need for further review, documentation, or justification. Only peer review can determine whether such variations are appropriate. The use of Screening Tools alone for utilization review or as the basis to deny reimbursement for health services is inappropriate.

It is important to understand that Screening Tools are particularly useful in screening cases of morbidity and mortality. However, Screening Tools that address procedures or diagnoses lack specificity or sensitivity, or both; consequently, their usefulness is limited. In using Screening Tools that address procedures or diagnoses, many charts fail the screen, but relatively few, after physician review, are determined to represent quality issues.

Purpose

The purpose of this Screening Tool is to identify those cases that may require physician review because they fail to meet the listed criteria for screening patients hospitalized for preeclampsia. Identified cases may require physician review for QI purposes.

Diagnosis

Preeclampsia (Mild) (ICD-9-CM Code 642.43 if affecting management of mother antepartum)

Bibliography

American College of Obstetricians and Gynecologists. Hypertension in pregnancy. ACOG Technical Bulletin 219. Washington, DC: ACOG, 1996

Screening Criteria

Hospitalization for Preeclampsia

Unless otherwise indicated, any time an unshaded box is checked, the chart should be referred for physician review.

Were the following documented in the medical record?	Yes	No
1. Patient history of (a *or* b *and* c):		
a. Sustained systolic blood pressure greater than 140 mm Hg*	■	❐
b. Sustained diastolic blood pressure greater than 90 mm Hg*		
c. Proteinuria	■	❐
2. Bed rest	■	❐
3. Monitoring including:		
a. Blood pressure at least three times per day	■	❐
b. Daily weight	■	❐
c. Urine protein testing	■	❐
d. Liver and renal functions and platelet count	■	❐
e. Recorded fetal heart tones at least daily	■	❐

* At least two readings 6 hours apart

STATEMENT REGARDING THE USE OF SCREENING TOOLS. The American College of Obstetricians and Gynecologists (ACOG), through the Committee on Quality Assessment, develops Screening Tools to assist in retrospective chart review to evaluate quality of patient care. They are based primarily on ACOG publications and consensus opinions and do not necessarily mention all acceptable clinical approaches. Departments of obstetrics and gynecology may modify these criteria to reflect local practice. The purpose of Screening Tools is to aid in identifying practice variances that might indicate the need for further review, documentation, or justification. Only peer review can determine whether such variations are appropriate. The use of Screening Tools alone for utilization review or as the basis to deny reimbursement for health services is inappropriate. It is important to understand that Screening Tools are particularly useful in screening cases of morbidity and mortality. However, Screening Tools that address procedures or diagnoses lack specificity or sensitivity, or both; consequently, their usefulness is limited. In using Screening Tools that address procedures or diagnoses, many charts fail the screen, but relatively few, after physician review, are determined to represent quality issues.

ACOG SCREENING TOOL

POSTTERM PREGNANCY

STATEMENT REGARDING THE USE OF SCREENING TOOLS. The American College of Obstetricians and Gynecologists (ACOG), through the Committee on Quality Assessment, develops Screening Tools to assist in retrospective chart review to evaluate quality of patient care. They are based primarily on ACOG publications and consensus opinions and do not necessarily mention all acceptable clinical approaches. Departments of obstetrics and gynecology may modify these criteria to reflect local practice. The purpose of Screening Tools is to aid in identifying practice variances that might indicate the need for further review, documentation, or justification. Only peer review can determine whether such variations are appropriate. The use of Screening Tools alone for utilization review or as the basis to deny reimbursement for health services is inappropriate.

It is important to understand that Screening Tools are particularly useful in screening cases of morbidity and mortality. However, Screening Tools that address procedures or diagnoses lack specificity or sensitivity, or both; consequently, their usefulness is limited. In using Screening Tools that address procedures or diagnoses, many charts fail the screen, but relatively few, after physician review, are determined to represent quality issues.

Purpose

The purpose of this Screening Tool is to identify those cases that may require physician review because they fail to meet the listed criteria for screening patients with postterm pregnancy (ie, a pregnancy that has advanced beyond 42 weeks of gestation) (ICD-9-CM Code 645.XX). Identified cases may require physician review for QI purposes.

Bibliography

American College of Obstetricians and Gynecologists. Management of postterm pregnancy. ACOG Practice Patterns 6. Washington, DC: ACOG, 1997

Screening Criteria

Postterm Pregnancy

Unless otherwise indicated, any time an unshaded box is checked, the chart should be referred for physician review.

Were the following documented in the medical record?   Yes   No

1. Length of gestation equal to or exceeding 42 weeks (294 days) based on any of the following: ■   ☐
   a. Length of gestation from an initial clinical examination early in pregnancy (uterine size should be compatible with last menstrual period)
   b. Ultrasonography performed at or before 20 weeks of gestation
   c. Known date of conception associated with infertility treatment

2. Antepartum management (a *and* b *and* [c *or* d *or* e]):
   a. Antepartum fetal surveillance performed by 42 weeks of gestation using standard protocols (eg, nonstress test, contraction stress test, biophysical profile, or modified biophysical profile [amniotic fluid and nonstress test])   ■   ☐
   b. Patient counseled to contact provider or proceed to labor and delivery if any of the following occurs   ■   ☐
      (1) Reduction in fetal movement
      (2) Onset of regular uterine contractions
      (3) Rupture of membranes
   c. Delivery for nonreassuring antepartum testing results   ■   ☐
   d. Induction of labor at 42 weeks of gestation if favorable cervix, unless contraindicated
   e. If 42 weeks of gestation and unfavorable cervix, use of cervical ripening agents unless contraindicated

3. Intrapartum management:
   a. Fetal heart monitoring performed in labor   ■   ☐
   b. In the presence of meconium, upper airway suctioned before delivery of fetal thorax   ■   ☐

STATEMENT REGARDING THE USE OF SCREENING TOOLS. The American College of Obstetricians and Gynecologists (ACOG), through the Committee on Quality Assessment, develops Screening Tools to assist in retrospective chart review to evaluate quality of patient care. They are based primarily on ACOG publications and consensus opinions and do not necessarily mention all acceptable clinical approaches. Departments of obstetrics and gynecology may modify these criteria to reflect local practice. The purpose of Screening Tools is to aid in identifying practice variances that might indicate the need for further review, documentation, or justification. Only peer review can determine whether such variations are appropriate. The use of Screening Tools alone for utilization review or as the basis to deny reimbursement for health services is inappropriate. It is important to understand that Screening Tools are particularly useful in screening cases of morbidity and mortality. However, Screening Tools that address procedures or diagnoses lack specificity or sensitivity, or both; consequently, their usefulness is limited. In using Screening Tools that address procedures or diagnoses, many charts fail the screen, but relatively few, after physician review, are determined to represent quality issues.

ACOG SCREENING TOOL

REPEAT CESAREAN DELIVERY

STATEMENT REGARDING THE USE OF SCREENING TOOLS. The American College of Obstetricians and Gynecologists (ACOG), through the Committee on Quality Assessment, develops Screening Tools to assist in retrospective chart review to evaluate quality of patient care. They are based primarily on ACOG publications and consensus opinions and do not necessarily mention all acceptable clinical approaches. Departments of obstetrics and gynecology may modify these criteria to reflect local practice. The purpose of Screening Tools is to aid in identifying practice variances that might indicate the need for further review, documentation, or justification. Only peer review can determine whether such variations are appropriate. The use of Screening Tools alone for utilization review or as the basis to deny reimbursement for health services is inappropriate.

It is important to understand that Screening Tools are particularly useful in screening cases of morbidity and mortality. However, Screening Tools that address procedures or diagnoses lack specificity or sensitivity, or both; consequently, their usefulness is limited. In using Screening Tools that address procedures or diagnoses, many charts fail the screen, but relatively few, after physician review, are determined to represent quality issues.

Purpose

The purpose of this Screening Tool is to identify those cases that may require physician review because they fail to meet the listed criteria for screening patients having an elective repeat cesarean delivery. Identified cases may require physician review for QI purposes.

Procedure

Cesarean delivery (ICD-9-CM Procedural Codes 74.0 or 74.1) (**CPT* Codes 59510** or **59618**) and previous cesarean delivery (ICD-9-CM Code 654.21)

*CPT only © 1999 American Medical Association. All rights reserved.

Bibliography

American College of Obstetricians and Gynecologists. Vaginal delivery after previous cesarean delivery. ACOG Practice Bulletin 5. Washington, DC: ACOG, 1999

American College of Obstetricians and Gynecologists. Assessment of fetal lung maturity. ACOG Educational Bulletin 230. Washington, DC: ACOG, 1996

Screening Criteria

Repeat Cesarean Delivery

Unless otherwise indicated, any time an unshaded box is checked, the chart should be referred for physician review.

Were the following documented in the medical record?   Yes   No

1. Fetal pulmonary maturity as documented by any of the following: ■   ❑
   a. Fetal heart tones for 20 weeks by nonelectronic fetoscope or for 30 weeks by Doppler
   b. Serum or urine hCG pregnancy test result found to be positive by a reliable laboratory at least 36 weeks previously
   c. Ultrasound measurement before 20 weeks confirming gestational age of greater than or equal to 39 weeks
   d. Amniocentesis that demonstrates fetal lung maturity

2. Previous uterine scar and, after appropriate counseling, patient declines attempt at vaginal birth   ■   ❑

STATEMENT REGARDING THE USE OF SCREENING TOOLS. The American College of Obstetricians and Gynecologists (ACOG), through the Committee on Quality Assessment, develops Screening Tools to assist in retrospective chart review to evaluate quality of patient care. They are based primarily on ACOG publications and consensus opinions and do not necessarily mention all acceptable clinical approaches. Departments of obstetrics and gynecology may modify these criteria to reflect local practice. The purpose of Screening Tools is to aid in identifying practice variances that might indicate the need for further review, documentation, or justification. Only peer review can determine whether such variations are appropriate. The use of Screening Tools alone for utilization review or as the basis to deny reimbursement for health services is inappropriate. It is important to understand that Screening Tools are particularly useful in screening cases of morbidity and mortality. However, Screening Tools that address procedures or diagnoses lack specificity or sensitivity, or both; consequently, their usefulness is limited. In using Screening Tools that address procedures or diagnoses, many charts fail the screen, but relatively few, after physician review, are determined to represent quality issues.

ACOG Screening Tool

Abdominal Hysterectomy with or Without Adnexectomy for Endometriosis

Statement Regarding the Use of Screening Tools. The American College of Obstetricians and Gynecologists (ACOG), through the Committee on Quality Assessment, develops Screening Tools to assist in retrospective chart review to evaluate quality of patient care. They are based primarily on ACOG publications and consensus opinions and do not necessarily mention all acceptable clinical approaches. Departments of obstetrics and gynecology may modify these criteria to reflect local practice. The purpose of Screening Tools is to aid in identifying practice variances that might indicate the need for further review, documentation, or justification. Only peer review can determine whether such variations are appropriate. The use of Screening Tools alone for utilization review or as the basis to deny reimbursement for health services is inappropriate.

It is important to understand that Screening Tools are particularly useful in screening cases of morbidity and mortality. However, Screening Tools that address procedures or diagnoses lack specificity or sensitivity, or both; consequently, their usefulness is limited. In using Screening Tools that address procedures or diagnoses, many charts fail the screen, but relatively few, after physician review, are determined to represent quality issues.

Purpose

The purpose of this Screening Tool is to identify those cases that may require physician review because they fail to meet the listed criteria for screening patients undergoing abdominal hysterectomy with or without adnexectomy for endometriosis. Identified cases may require physician review for QI purposes.

Procedure

Abdominal hysterectomy with or without adnexectomy for endometriosis (ICD-9-CM Procedural Codes 65.3, 65.4, 65.5, 65.6, 68.4) (**CPT* Code 58150**)

Indication

Endometriosis (ICD-9-CM Codes 617.0–617.9)

Bibliography

American College of Obstetricians and Gynecologists. Medical management of endometriosis. ACOG Practice Bulletin 11. Washington, DC: ACOG, 1999

---

*CPT only © 1999 American Medical Association. All rights reserved.

Screening Criteria

Abdominal Hysterectomy with or Without Adnexectomy for Endometriosis

Unless otherwise indicated, any time an unshaded box is checked, the chart should be referred for physician review.

Were the following documented in the medical record?	Yes	No
1. Patient history of (a *and* b *and* [c *or* d *or* e])		
a. Prior detailed operative description or histologic diagnosis of endometriosis	■	❏
b. Presence of pain for more than 6 months with negative effect on patient's quality of life	■	❏
c. Failure of conservative measures to control significant symptoms	■	❏
d. Presence of persistent, significant adnexal mass		
e. Significant involvement of other organ systems, eg, ureteral or intestinal obstruction		
2. Failure of a therapeutic trial with one or more of the following or contraindications to use	■	❏
a. Oral contraceptives		
b. Nonsteroidal antiinflammatory drugs		
c. Agents for inducing amenorrhea (eg, GnRH analogs or danazol)		
3. Nonmalignant cervical cytology	■	❏
4. Results of endometrial sample or dilation and curettage when abnormal uterine bleeding is present	■	❏
5. Negative preoperative pregnancy test unless patient is postmenopausal	■	❏
6. Patient desire for definitive surgical therapy	■	❏
7. Antibiotic prophylaxis administered preoperatively	■	❏

Statement Regarding the Use of Screening Tools. The American College of Obstetricians and Gynecologists (ACOG), through the Committee on Quality Assessment, develops Screening Tools to assist in retrospective chart review to evaluate quality of patient care. They are based primarily on ACOG publications and consensus opinions and do not necessarily mention all acceptable clinical approaches. Departments of obstetrics and gynecology may modify these criteria to reflect local practice. The purpose of Screening Tools is to aid in identifying practice variances that might indicate the need for further review, documentation, or justification. Only peer review can determine whether such variations are appropriate. The use of Screening Tools alone for utilization review or as the basis to deny reimbursement for health services is inappropriate. It is important to understand that Screening Tools are particularly useful in screening cases of morbidity and mortality. However, Screening Tools that address procedures or diagnoses lack specificity or sensitivity, or both; consequently, their usefulness is limited. In using Screening Tools that address procedures or diagnoses, many charts fail the screen, but relatively few, after physician review, are determined to represent quality issues.

ACOG Screening Tool

Diagnostic Laparoscopy for Acute Pelvic Pain

Statement Regarding the Use of Screening Tools. The American College of Obstetricians and Gynecologists (ACOG), through the Committee on Quality Assessment, develops Screening Tools to assist in retrospective chart review to evaluate quality of patient care. They are based primarily on ACOG publications and consensus opinions and do not necessarily mention all acceptable clinical approaches. Departments of obstetrics and gynecology may modify these criteria to reflect local practice. The purpose of Screening Tools is to aid in identifying practice variances that might indicate the need for further review, documentation, or justification. Only peer review can determine whether such variations are appropriate. The use of Screening Tools alone for utilization review or as the basis to deny reimbursement for health services is inappropriate.

It is important to understand that Screening Tools are particularly useful in screening cases of morbidity and mortality. However, Screening Tools that address procedures or diagnoses lack specificity or sensitivity, or both; consequently, their usefulness is limited. In using Screening Tools that address procedures or diagnoses, many charts fail the screen, but relatively few, after physician review, are determined to represent quality issues.

Purpose

The purpose of this Screening Tool is to identify those cases that may require physician review because they fail to meet the listed criteria for screening patients undergoing diagnostic laparoscopy performed for acute pelvic pain (onset of <72 hours before surgery). Identified cases may require physician review for QI purposes.

Procedure

Diagnostic laparoscopy (ICD-9-CM Procedural Code 54.21) (**CPT* Code 49320**) for acute pelvic pain

Indication

Pelvic pain (ICD-9-CM 625.9) of recent onset

*CPT only © 1999 American Medical Association. All rights reserved.

Screening Criteria
Diagnostic Laparoscopy for Acute Pelvic Pain

Unless otherwise indicated, any time an unshaded box is checked, the chart should be referred for physician review.

	Yes	No
1. Were the following documented in the medical record?		
a. Onset, severity, duration, and location of pain	■	☐
b. Physical examination confirming the presence of abdominal or pelvic tenderness	■	☐
c. Urinalysis, including microscopic examination	■	☐
d. Pregnancy test for patients of reproductive age	■	☐
e. Last normal menstrual period	■	☐
f. Complete blood count with differential	■	☐
g. Vital signs (blood pressure, pulse, and temperature)	■	☐
2. Was a laparotomy performed?	☐	■

STATEMENT REGARDING THE USE OF SCREENING TOOLS. The American College of Obstetricians and Gynecologists (ACOG), through the Committee on Quality Assessment, develops Screening Tools to assist in retrospective chart review to evaluate quality of patient care. They are based primarily on ACOG publications and consensus opinions and do not necessarily mention all acceptable clinical approaches. Departments of obstetrics and gynecology may modify these criteria to reflect local practice. The purpose of Screening Tools is to aid in identifying practice variances that might indicate the need for further review, documentation, or justification. Only peer review can determine whether such variations are appropriate. The use of Screening Tools alone for utilization review or as the basis to deny reimbursement for health services is inappropriate. It is important to understand that Screening Tools are particularly useful in screening cases of morbidity and mortality. However, Screening Tools that address procedures or diagnoses lack specificity or sensitivity, or both; consequently, their usefulness is limited. In using Screening Tools that address procedures or diagnoses, many charts fail the screen, but relatively few, after physician review, are determined to represent quality issues.

ACOG SCREENING TOOL

ECTOPIC PREGNANCY, RUPTURED
Ambulatory Care Sensitive Indicator*

STATEMENT REGARDING THE USE OF SCREENING TOOLS. The American College of Obstetricians and Gynecologists (ACOG), through the Committee on Quality Assessment, develops Screening Tools to assist in retrospective chart review to evaluate quality of patient care. They are based primarily on ACOG publications and consensus opinions and do not necessarily mention all acceptable clinical approaches. Departments of obstetrics and gynecology may modify these criteria to reflect local practice. The purpose of Screening Tools is to aid in identifying practice variances that might indicate the need for further review, documentation, or justification. Only peer review can determine whether such variations are appropriate. The use of Screening Tools alone for utilization review or as the basis to deny reimbursement for health services is inappropriate.

It is important to understand that Screening Tools are particularly useful in screening cases of morbidity and mortality. However, Screening Tools that address procedures or diagnoses lack specificity or sensitivity, or both; consequently, their usefulness is limited. In using Screening Tools that address procedures or diagnoses, many charts fail the screen, but relatively few, after physician review, are determined to represent quality issues.

Purpose

The purpose of this Screening Tool is to identify those cases that may require physician review because they fail to meet the listed criteria for screening patients with a ruptured ectopic pregnancy. Identified cases may require physician review for QI purposes.

Procedure

Removal of extratubal ectopic pregnancy (ICD-9-CM Procedural Code 74.3) (CPT† Codes 59120, 59121, 59130, 59135, 59136, 59140, 59150, 59151)

Indications

Presence of ruptured ectopic pregnancy (ICD-9-CM Codes 633.0X–633.9X)

Bibliography

American College of Obstetricians and Gynecologists. Medical management of tubal pregnancy. ACOG Practice Bulletin 3. Washington, DC: ACOG, 1998

---

* Used to help determine the quality of care that was provided, in an ambulatory setting, which may have contributed to an adverse outcome

†CPT only © 1999 American Medical Association. All rights reserved.

Screening Criteria

Ectopic Pregnancy, Ruptured

Unless otherwise indicated, any time an unshaded box is checked, the chart should be referred for physician review.

Were the following documented in the hospital medical record? | Yes | No

1. Patient history of (a *and* b *and* [c *or* d])
   a. Ruptured ectopic pregnancy ■ ☐
   b. Prior outpatient care related to this episode ■ ☐
   c. Prior related abdominal or pelvic pain ■ ☐
   d. Prior and related abnormal vaginal bleeding

Were the following documented in the ambulatory care record?

1. Last menstrual period ■ ☐

2. Inquiry regarding abnormal uterine bleeding ■ ☐

3. Inquiry regarding abdominal or pelvic pain ■ ☐

4. Blood pressure and pulse ■ ☐

5. Abdominal and pelvic examination ■ ☐

6. Results of pregnancy test ■ ☐

7. Appointment for follow-up care ■ ☐

8. For patients who had a positive pregnancy test result documented in the ambulatory setting, did the record indicate the following plan?
   a. Ultrasonography at appropriate discriminatory levels of β-hCG* ■ ☐
   b. Patient counseling regarding ectopic precautions ■ ☐
   c. Serial quantitative β-hCG level ■ ☐

*As defined by the hospital

STATEMENT REGARDING THE USE OF SCREENING TOOLS. The American College of Obstetricians and Gynecologists (ACOG), through the Committee on Quality Assessment, develops Screening Tools to assist in retrospective chart review to evaluate quality of patient care. They are based primarily on ACOG publications and consensus opinions and do not necessarily mention all acceptable clinical approaches. Departments of obstetrics and gynecology may modify these criteria to reflect local practice. The purpose of Screening Tools is to aid in identifying practice variances that might indicate the need for further review, documentation, or justification. Only peer review can determine whether such variations are appropriate. The use of Screening Tools alone for utilization review or as the basis to deny reimbursement for health services is inappropriate. It is important to understand that Screening Tools are particularly useful in screening cases of morbidity and mortality. However, Screening Tools that address procedures or diagnoses lack specificity or sensitivity, or both; consequently, their usefulness is limited. In using Screening Tools that address procedures or diagnoses, many charts fail the screen, but relatively few, after physician review, are determined to represent quality issues.

ACOG Screening Tool

Endometrial Ablation

Statement Regarding the Use of Screening Tools. The American College of Obstetricians and Gynecologists (ACOG), through the Committee on Quality Assessment, develops Screening Tools to assist in retrospective chart review to evaluate quality of patient care. They are based primarily on ACOG publications and consensus opinions and do not necessarily mention all acceptable clinical approaches. Departments of obstetrics and gynecology may modify these criteria to reflect local practice. The purpose of Screening Tools is to aid in identifying practice variances that might indicate the need for further review, documentation, or justification. Only peer review can determine whether such variations are appropriate. The use of Screening Tools alone for utilization review or as the basis to deny reimbursement for health services is inappropriate.

It is important to understand that Screening Tools are particularly useful in screening cases of morbidity and mortality. However, Screening Tools that address procedures or diagnoses lack specificity or sensitivity, or both; consequently, their usefulness is limited. In using Screening Tools that address procedures or diagnoses, many charts fail the screen, but relatively few, after physician review, are determined to represent quality issues.

Purpose

The purpose of this Screening Tool is to identify those cases that may require physician review because they fail to meet the listed criteria for screening patients undergoing endometrial ablation for abnormal uterine bleeding. Identified cases may require physician review for QI purposes.

Procedure

Endometrial ablation for abnormal uterine bleeding in women of reproductive age (**CPT* Code 58563**) (ICD-9-CM Codes 626.2, 626.4, 626.6, 626.8)

*CPT only © 1999 American Medical Association. All rights reserved.

Bibliography

American College of Obstetricians and Gynecologists. Management of anovulatory bleeding. ACOG Practice Bulletin 14. Washington, DC: ACOG, 2000

Screening Criteria

Endometrial Ablation

Unless otherwise indicated, any time an unshaded box is checked, the chart should be referred for physician review.

Were the following documented in the medical record?	Yes	No
1. Patient history of		
a. Excessive uterine bleeding evidenced by either (1 *or* 2)	■	❏
(1) Profuse bleeding lasting more than 7 days or repetitive periods at less than 21-day intervals		
(2) Anemia due to acute or chronic blood loss		
b. Failure of hormonal treatment or contraindication to hormonal use	■	❏
c. No current medication use that may cause bleeding, or contraindication to stopping those medications	■	❏
d. Assessment for absence of endometrial malignancy	■	❏
e. No evidence of remediable pathology by (1 *or* 2 *or* 3)	■	❏
(1) Sonohysterogram		
(2) Hysteroscopy		
(3) Hysterosalpingogram		
2. Nonmalignant cervical cytology	■	❏
3. Negative preoperative pregnancy test result unless patient is postmenopausal	■	❏
4. Absence of abnormal coagulation studies	■	❏
5. Absence of malignancy or atypical hyperplasia on endometrial sampling	■	❏

STATEMENT REGARDING THE USE OF SCREENING TOOLS. The American College of Obstetricians and Gynecologists (ACOG), through the Committee on Quality Assessment, develops Screening Tools to assist in retrospective chart review to evaluate quality of patient care. They are based primarily on ACOG publications and consensus opinions and do not necessarily mention all acceptable clinical approaches. Departments of obstetrics and gynecology may modify these criteria to reflect local practice. The purpose of Screening Tools is to aid in identifying practice variances that might indicate the need for further review, documentation, or justification. Only peer review can determine whether such variations are appropriate. The use of Screening Tools alone for utilization review or as the basis to deny reimbursement for health services is inappropriate. It is important to understand that Screening Tools are particularly useful in screening cases of morbidity and mortality. However, Screening Tools that address procedures or diagnoses lack specificity or sensitivity, or both; consequently, their usefulness is limited. In using Screening Tools that address procedures or diagnoses, many charts fail the screen, but relatively few, after physician review, are determined to represent quality issues.

ACOG SCREENING TOOL

FEMALE STERILIZATION BY TUBAL INTERRUPTION

STATEMENT REGARDING THE USE OF SCREENING TOOLS. The American College of Obstetricians and Gynecologists (ACOG), through the Committee on Quality Assessment, develops Screening Tools to assist in retrospective chart review to evaluate quality of patient care. They are based primarily on ACOG publications and consensus opinions and do not necessarily mention all acceptable clinical approaches. Departments of obstetrics and gynecology may modify these criteria to reflect local practice. The purpose of Screening Tools is to aid in identifying practice variances that might indicate the need for further review, documentation, or justification. Only peer review can determine whether such variations are appropriate. The use of Screening Tools alone for utilization review or as the basis to deny reimbursement for health services is inappropriate.

It is important to understand that Screening Tools are particularly useful in screening cases of morbidity and mortality. However, Screening Tools that address procedures or diagnoses lack specificity or sensitivity, or both; consequently, their usefulness is limited. In using Screening Tools that address procedures or diagnoses, many charts fail the screen, but relatively few, after physician review, are determined to represent quality issues.

Purpose

The purpose of this Screening Tool is to identify those cases that may require physician review because they fail to meet the listed criteria for screening patients undergoing female sterilization by tubal interruption. Identified cases may require physician review for QI purposes.

Procedure

Female sterilization by tubal interruption, all methods (ICD-9 Procedural Codes 66.21–66.29) (**CPT* Codes 58600, 58605, 58611, 58615, 58670, 58671, and 58700**)

Indication

Undesired fertility (ICD-9-CM Code V25.2)

Bibliography

American College of Obstetricians and Gynecologists. Sterilization. ACOG Technical Bulletin 222. Washington, DC: ACOG, 1996

American College of Obstetricians and Gynecologists. Sterilization of women, including those with mental disabilities. ACOG Committee Opinion 216. Washington, DC: ACOG, 1999

*CPT only © 1999 American Medical Association. All rights reserved.

Screening Criteria

Female Sterilization by Tubal Interruption

Unless otherwise indicated, any time an unshaded box is checked, the chart should be referred for physician review.

Were the following documented in the medical record before the procedure?	Yes	No
1. Patient request for permanent sterilization	■	☐
2. Informed consent in compliance with appropriate state and federal regulations, including the following:		
a. Alternate forms of contraception	■	☐
b. Specific procedure to be performed, including failure rate	■	☐
c. Potential for ectopic as well as intrauterine pregnancy	■	☐
d. Permanence of procedure	■	☐
3. Last menstrual period*	■	☐
4. Negative preoperative pregnancy test*	■	☐

* This is not appropriate for puerperal sterilization or procedures performed in conjunction with abortion (spontaneous or elective).

STATEMENT REGARDING THE USE OF SCREENING TOOLS. The American College of Obstetricians and Gynecologists (ACOG), through the Committee on Quality Assessment, develops Screening Tools to assist in retrospective chart review to evaluate quality of patient care. They are based primarily on ACOG publications and consensus opinions and do not necessarily mention all acceptable clinical approaches. Departments of obstetrics and gynecology may modify these criteria to reflect local practice. The purpose of Screening Tools is to aid in identifying practice variances that might indicate the need for further review, documentation, or justification. Only peer review can determine whether such variations are appropriate. The use of Screening Tools alone for utilization review or as the basis to deny reimbursement for health services is inappropriate. It is important to understand that Screening Tools are particularly useful in screening cases of morbidity and mortality. However, Screening Tools that address procedures or diagnoses lack specificity or sensitivity, or both; consequently, their usefulness is limited. In using Screening Tools that address procedures or diagnoses, many charts fail the screen, but relatively few, after physician review, are determined to represent quality issues.

ACOG Screening Tool

Hysterectomy for Abnormal Uterine Bleeding in Premenopausal Women

Statement Regarding the Use of Screening Tools. The American College of Obstetricians and Gynecologists (ACOG), through the Committee on Quality Assessment, develops Screening Tools to assist in retrospective chart review to evaluate quality of patient care. They are based primarily on ACOG publications and consensus opinions and do not necessarily mention all acceptable clinical approaches. Departments of obstetrics and gynecology may modify these criteria to reflect local practice. The purpose of Screening Tools is to aid in identifying practice variances that might indicate the need for further review, documentation, or justification. Only peer review can determine whether such variations are appropriate. The use of Screening Tools alone for utilization review or as the basis to deny reimbursement for health services is inappropriate.

It is important to understand that Screening Tools are particularly useful in screening cases of morbidity and mortality. However, Screening Tools that address procedures or diagnoses lack specificity or sensitivity, or both; consequently, their usefulness is limited. In using Screening Tools that address procedures or diagnoses, many charts fail the screen, but relatively few, after physician review, are determined to represent quality issues.

Purpose

The purpose of this Screening Tool is to identify those cases that may require physician review because they fail to meet the listed criteria for screening patients undergoing hysterectomy for abnormal uterine bleeding. Identified cases may require physician review for QI purposes.

Procedure

Hysterectomy, abdominal (ICD-9 Procedural Code 68.4) (**CPT* Code 58150**) or vaginal (68.5) (**CPT Codes 58260, 58262, or 58550**) for abnormal uterine bleeding.

Indication

Abnormal uterine bleeding in premenopausal women (ICD-9-CM Code 626 all, except 626.0, 626.1, 626.3, 626.5, 626.7) (Other diagnoses that also should be evaluated according to these criteria include menorrhagia [626.2, 627.0], hypermenorrhea [626.2], dysfunctional uterine bleeding, menometrorrhagia [626.2], and polymenorrhea [626.2].)

---

*CPT only © 1999 American Medical Association. All rights reserved.

Screening Criteria

Hysterectomy for Abnormal Uterine Bleeding in Premenopausal Women

Unless otherwise indicated, any time an unshaded box is checked, the chart should be referred for physician review.

Were the following documented in the medical record before the procedure?   Yes   No

1. Patient history of:
   a. Excessive uterine bleeding evidence by either (1 *or* 2):   ■   ❐
      (1) Profuse bleeding lasting more than 7 days or repetitive periods at less than 21-day intervals
      (2) Anemia due to acute or chronic blood loss
   b. Failure of hormonal treatment or contraindication to hormone use   ■   ❐
   c. No current medication use that may cause bleeding, or contraindication to stopping those medications   ■   ❐
   d. Endometrial sampling performed   ■   ❐
   e. No evidence of remediable pathology by (1 *or* 2 *or* 3)   ■   ❐
      (1) Sonohysterogram
      (2) Hysteroscopy
      (3) Hysterosalpingogram

2. Negative preoperative pregnancy test result unless patient is postmenopausal   ■   ❐

3. Assessment of surgical risk from anemia and need for treatment   ■   ❐

4. Consideration of alternative therapeutic approaches (eg, endometrial ablation)   ■   ❐

5. Antibiotic prophylaxis administered preoperatively   ■   ❐

STATEMENT REGARDING THE USE OF SCREENING TOOLS. The American College of Obstetricians and Gynecologists (ACOG), through the Committee on Quality Assessment, develops Screening Tools to assist in retrospective chart review to evaluate quality of patient care. They are based primarily on ACOG publications and consensus opinions and do not necessarily mention all acceptable clinical approaches. Departments of obstetrics and gynecology may modify these criteria to reflect local practice. The purpose of Screening Tools is to aid in identifying practice variances that might indicate the need for further review, documentation, or justification. Only peer review can determine whether such variations are appropriate. The use of Screening Tools alone for utilization review or as the basis to deny reimbursement for health services is inappropriate. It is important to understand that Screening Tools are particularly useful in screening cases of morbidity and mortality. However, Screening Tools that address procedures or diagnoses lack specificity or sensitivity, or both; consequently, their usefulness is limited. In using Screening Tools that address procedures or diagnoses, many charts fail the screen, but relatively few, after physician review, are determined to represent quality issues.

ACOG Screening Tool

Hysterectomy for Leiomyomata

STATEMENT REGARDING THE USE OF SCREENING TOOLS. The American College of Obstetricians and Gynecologists (ACOG), through the Committee on Quality Assessment, develops Screening Tools to assist in retrospective chart review to evaluate quality of patient care. They are based primarily on ACOG publications and consensus opinions and do not necessarily mention all acceptable clinical approaches. Departments of obstetrics and gynecology may modify these criteria to reflect local practice. The purpose of Screening Tools is to aid in identifying practice variances that might indicate the need for further review, documentation, or justification. Only peer review can determine whether such variations are appropriate. The use of Screening Tools alone for utilization review or as the basis to deny reimbursement for health services is inappropriate.

It is important to understand that Screening Tools are particularly useful in screening cases of morbidity and mortality. However, Screening Tools that address procedures or diagnoses lack specificity or sensitivity, or both; consequently, their usefulness is limited. In using Screening Tools that address procedures or diagnoses, many charts fail the screen, but relatively few, after physician review, are determined to represent quality issues.

Purpose

The purpose of this Screening Tool is to identify those cases that may require physician review because they fail to meet the listed criteria for screening patients undergoing hysterectomy for the indication leiomyomata uteri. Identified cases may require physician review for QI purposes.

Procedure

Hysterectomy, abdominal (ICD-9-CM Procedural Code 68.4) (**CPT* Code 58150**) or vaginal (68.51 or 68.59) (**CPT Codes 58260, 58262**), or laparoscopically assisted (**CPT Code 58550**)

Indication

Leiomyomata for patients not desiring to retain uterus (ICD-9-CM Codes 218.0 – 218.9)

Bibliography

American College of Obstetricians and Gynecologists. Surgical alternatives to hysterectomy in the management of leiomyomas. ACOG Practice Bulletin 16. Washington, DC: ACOG, 2000

*CPT only © 1999 American Medical Association. All rights reserved.

Screening Criteria
Hysterectomy for Leiomyomata

Unless otherwise indicated, any time an unshaded box is checked, the chart should be referred for physician review.

Were the following documented in the medical record?	Yes	No
1. Patient history of (either a *or* b *or* c):	■	☐
a. Leiomyomata enlarging the uterus to a size of 12 weeks or greater gestation and are a concern to the patient		
b. Leiomyomata as probable cause of excessive uterine bleeding evidenced by either (1 *or* 2):		
(1) Profuse bleeding lasting more than 7 days or repetitive periods at less than 21-day intervals		
(2) Anemia due to acute or chronic blood loss		
c. Pelvic discomfort caused by myomata (1 *or* 2 *or* 3)	■	☐
(1) Chronic lower abdominal, pelvic, or low back pressure		
(2) Bladder dysfunction not due to urinary tract disorder or disease		
(3) Rectal pressure and bowel dysfunction not related to bowel disorder or disease		
2. Discussion of risks, benefits, and options to planned procedure	■	☐
3. Nonmalignant cervical cytology	■	☐
4. Assessment for absence of endometrial malignancy if pattern of bleeding is not characteristic of leiomyomata (ie, if abnormal bleeding is anything other than menorrhagia)	■	☐
5. Assessment of anemia if heavy bleeding is present	■	☐
6. Negative preoperative pregnancy test unless patient is postmenopausal	■	☐
7. Anovulation eliminated as a cause of abnormal uterine bleeding, if present	■	☐
8. Antibiotic prophylaxis administered preoperatively	■	☐

STATEMENT REGARDING THE USE OF SCREENING TOOLS. The American College of Obstetricians and Gynecologists (ACOG), through the Committee on Quality Assessment, develops Screening Tools to assist in retrospective chart review to evaluate quality of patient care. They are based primarily on ACOG publications and consensus opinions and do not necessarily mention all acceptable clinical approaches. Departments of obstetrics and gynecology may modify these criteria to reflect local practice. The purpose of Screening Tools is to aid in identifying practice variances that might indicate the need for further review, documentation, or justification. Only peer review can determine whether such variations are appropriate. The use of Screening Tools alone for utilization review or as the basis to deny reimbursement for health services is inappropriate. It is important to understand that Screening Tools are particularly useful in screening cases of morbidity and mortality. However, Screening Tools that address procedures or diagnoses lack specificity or sensitivity, or both; consequently, their usefulness is limited. In using Screening Tools that address procedures or diagnoses, many charts fail the screen, but relatively few, after physician review, are determined to represent quality issues.

ACOG Screening Tool

Hysterectomy for Pelvic Organ Prolapse

Statement Regarding the Use of Screening Tools. The American College of Obstetricians and Gynecologists (ACOG), through the Committee on Quality Assessment, develops Screening Tools to assist in retrospective chart review to evaluate quality of patient care. They are based primarily on ACOG publications and consensus opinions and do not necessarily mention all acceptable clinical approaches. Departments of obstetrics and gynecology may modify these criteria to reflect local practice. The purpose of Screening Tools is to aid in identifying practice variances that might indicate the need for further review, documentation, or justification. Only peer review can determine whether such variations are appropriate. The use of Screening Tools alone for utilization review or as the basis to deny reimbursement for health services is inappropriate.

It is important to understand that Screening Tools are particularly useful in screening cases of morbidity and mortality. However, Screening Tools that address procedures or diagnoses lack specificity or sensitivity, or both; consequently, their usefulness is limited. In using Screening Tools that address procedures or diagnoses, many charts fail the screen, but relatively few, after physician review, are determined to represent quality issues.

Purpose

The purpose of this Screening Tool is to identify those cases that may require physician review because they fail to meet the listed criteria for screening patients undergoing hysterectomy for pelvic or vaginal wall relaxation (ICD-9-CM Procedural Codes 68.4, 68.5). Identified cases may require physician review for QI purposes.

Procedure

Hysterectomy, abdominal (ICD-9-CM Procedural Code 68.4) (**CPT* Code 58150**) or vaginal (ICD-9-CM Procedural Codes 68.51 or 68.59) (**CPT Codes 58260, 58262, 58550**) with repair of pelvic or vaginal wall relaxation defects (ICD-9-CM Procedural Codes 69.22, 69.29, 70.42, 70.50, or 70.8) (**CPT Codes 57240, 57250, 57260, 57265, 57268, 57270, 57280 or 57282, 57889, 58263, or 58270**)

Indications

Pelvic or vaginal wall relaxation—loss of support of the uterus or vagina (ICD-9-CM Codes 618 all). This procedure is indicated if symptoms are severe enough to justify the risks involved with surgery, if nonsurgical options have failed or have been rejected by the patient, or the patient is requesting relief.

Bibliography

American College of Obstetricians and Gynecologists. Pelvic organ prolapse. ACOG Technical Bulletin 214. Washington, DC: ACOG, 1995

*CPT only © 1999 American Medical Association. All rights reserved.

Screening Criteria

Hysterectomy for Pelvic Organ Prolapse

Unless otherwise indicated, any time an unshaded box is checked, the chart should be referred for physician review.

Were the following documented in the medical record?   Yes   No

1. Patient history of protrusions of the pelvic organs into or out of the vaginal wall   ■   ❏

2. Nonmalignant cervical cytology   ■   ❏

3. Endometrial assessment for malignancy, if indicated   ■   ❏

4. Physical examination, patient's symptoms, and pelvic support defects   ■   ❏

5. Antibiotic prophylaxis administered preoperatively   ■   ❏

6. Negative preoperative pregnancy test result unless patient is postmenopausal   ■   ❏

STATEMENT REGARDING THE USE OF SCREENING TOOLS. The American College of Obstetricians and Gynecologists (ACOG), through the Committee on Quality Assessment, develops Screening Tools to assist in retrospective chart review to evaluate quality of patient care. They are based primarily on ACOG publications and consensus opinions and do not necessarily mention all acceptable clinical approaches. Departments of obstetrics and gynecology may modify these criteria to reflect local practice. The purpose of Screening Tools is to aid in identifying practice variances that might indicate the need for further review, documentation, or justification. Only peer review can determine whether such variations are appropriate. The use of Screening Tools alone for utilization review or as the basis to deny reimbursement for health services is inappropriate. It is important to understand that Screening Tools are particularly useful in screening cases of morbidity and mortality. However, Screening Tools that address procedures or diagnoses lack specificity or sensitivity, or both; consequently, their usefulness is limited. In using Screening Tools that address procedures or diagnoses, many charts fail the screen, but relatively few, after physician review, are determined to represent quality issues.

ACOG SCREENING TOOL

HYSTERECTOMY PERFORMED FOR CHRONIC PELVIC PAIN IN THE ABSENCE OF SIGNIFICANT PATHOLOGY

STATEMENT REGARDING THE USE OF SCREENING TOOLS. The American College of Obstetricians and Gynecologists (ACOG), through the Committee on Quality Assessment, develops Screening Tools to assist in retrospective chart review to evaluate quality of patient care. They are based primarily on ACOG publications and consensus opinions and do not necessarily mention all acceptable clinical approaches. Departments of obstetrics and gynecology may modify these criteria to reflect local practice. The purpose of Screening Tools is to aid in identifying practice variances that might indicate the need for further review, documentation, or justification. Only peer review can determine whether such variations are appropriate. The use of Screening Tools alone for utilization review or as the basis to deny reimbursement for health services is inappropriate.

It is important to understand that Screening Tools are particularly useful in screening cases of morbidity and mortality. However, Screening Tools that address procedures or diagnoses lack specificity or sensitivity, or both; consequently, their usefulness is limited. In using Screening Tools that address procedures or diagnoses, many charts fail the screen, but relatively few, after physician review, are determined to represent quality issues.

Purpose

The purpose of this Screening Tool is to identify those cases that may require physician review because they fail to meet the listed criteria for screening patients undergoing hysterectomy for chronic pelvic pain in the absence of significant pelvic pathology. Identified cases may require physician review for QI purposes.

Procedure

Hysterectomy, abdominal (ICD-9-CM Procedural Code 68.4) **(CPT* Code 58150)** or vaginal (ICD-9-CM Procedural Code 68.5) **(CPT Codes 58260, 58262, or 58550)** for chronic pelvic pain

---

*CPT only © 1999 American Medical Association. All rights reserved.

Indication

Chronic pelvic pain in the absence of significant pathology (ICD-9-CM Code 625.9). Other diagnoses that also should be evaluated according to these criteria include pelvic congestion (625.5); pelvic varices (456.5); uterine retroversion (621.6); congenital anomalies (752.3); dysmenorrhea (625.3); mild endometriosis (617–617.9); minimal pelvic adhesions (614.6); broad ligament window (620.4); first-degree uterine prolapse (618–618.9); and mild adenomyosis (617.0)

Bibliography

American College of Obstetricians and Gynecologists. Chronic pelvic pain. ACOG Technical Bulletin 223. Washington, DC: ACOG, 1996

American College of Obstetricians and Gynecologists. Precis: Gynecology. Washington, DC: ACOG, 1999

Screening Criteria

Hysterectomy Performed for Chronic Pelvic Pain in the Absence of Significant Pathology

---

Unless otherwise indicated, any time an unshaded box is checked, the chart should be referred for physician review.

Were the following documented in the medical record?	Yes	No
1. Patient history of		
a. No remediable pathology found on laparoscopic examination	■	❏
b. Pain for more than 6 months with negative effect on patient's quality of life	■	❏
2. Failure of a therapeutic trial with one or more of the following or contraindication to use:	■	❏
a. Oral contraceptives		
b. Nonsteroidal antiinflammatory drugs		
c. Agents for inducing amenorrhea (eg, GnRH analogs or danazol)		
3. Evaluation of the following systems as possible sources of pelvic pain:		
a. Urinary	■	❏
b. Gastrointestinal	■	❏
c. Musculoskeletal	■	❏
4. Evaluation of the patient's psychologic and psychosexual status for nonsomatic cause	■	❏
5. Nonmalignant cervical cytology	■	❏
6. Results of endometrial biopsy or dilation and curettage when abnormal bleeding is present	■	❏
7. Negative preoperative pregnancy test unless patient is postmenopausal	■	❏
8. Antibiotic prophylaxis administered preoperatively	■	❏

STATEMENT REGARDING THE USE OF SCREENING TOOLS. The American College of Obstetricians and Gynecologists (ACOG), through the Committee on Quality Assessment, develops Screening Tools to assist in retrospective chart review to evaluate quality of patient care. They are based primarily on ACOG publications and consensus opinions and do not necessarily mention all acceptable clinical approaches. Departments of obstetrics and gynecology may modify these criteria to reflect local practice. The purpose of Screening Tools is to aid in identifying practice variances that might indicate the need for further review, documentation, or justification. Only peer review can determine whether such variations are appropriate. The use of Screening Tools alone for utilization review or as the basis to deny reimbursement for health services is inappropriate. It is important to understand that Screening Tools are particularly useful in screening cases of morbidity and mortality. However, Screening Tools that address procedures or diagnoses lack specificity or sensitivity, or both; consequently, their usefulness is limited. In using Screening Tools that address procedures or diagnoses, many charts fail the screen, but relatively few, after physician review, are determined to represent quality issues.

ACOG Screening Tool

Hysteroscopy for Abnormal Uterine Bleeding

Statement Regarding the Use of Screening Tools. The American College of Obstetricians and Gynecologists (ACOG), through the Committee on Quality Assessment, develops Screening Tools to assist in retrospective chart review to evaluate quality of patient care. They are based primarily on ACOG publications and consensus opinions and do not necessarily mention all acceptable clinical approaches. Departments of obstetrics and gynecology may modify these criteria to reflect local practice. The purpose of Screening Tools is to aid in identifying practice variances that might indicate the need for further review, documentation, or justification. Only peer review can determine whether such variations are appropriate. The use of Screening Tools alone for utilization review or as the basis to deny reimbursement for health services is inappropriate.

It is important to understand that Screening Tools are particularly useful in screening cases of morbidity and mortality. However, Screening Tools that address procedures or diagnoses lack specificity or sensitivity, or both; consequently, their usefulness is limited. In using Screening Tools that address procedures or diagnoses, many charts fail the screen, but relatively few, after physician review, are determined to represent quality issues.

Purpose

The purpose of this Screening Tool is to identify those cases that may require physician review because they fail to meet the listed criteria for screening patients undergoing diagnostic hysteroscopy for abnormal uterine bleeding. Identified cases may require physician review for QI purposes.

Procedure

Hysteroscopy, diagnostic, for abnormal uterine bleeding (**CPT* Code 58555**)

Indication

Abnormal uterine bleeding (ICD-9-CM Codes 626.2, 627.1)

Bibliography

American College of Obstetricians and Gynecologists. Hysteroscopy. ACOG Technical Bulletin 191. Washington, DC: ACOG, 1994

*CPT only © 1999 American Medical Association. All rights reserved.

Screening Criteria

Hysteroscopy for Abnormal Uterine Bleeding

Unless otherwise indicated, any time an unshaded box is checked, the chart should be referred for physician review.

Were the following documented in the medical record?   Yes   No

1. Patient history of either (a *or* b):   ■   ☐
    a. Postmenopausal bleeding
    b. All of the following
       (1) Failure to find cervical or uterine pathology that would cause abnormal bleeding
       (2) History of excessive uterine bleeding evidenced by profuse bleeding lasting more than
           7 days or repetitive periods at less than 21-day intervals
       (3) Failure of appropriate medical therapy

2. Pelvic examination   ■   ☐

3. Nonmalignant cervical cytology   ■   ☐

4. Negative preoperative pregnancy test result unless patient is postmenopausal   ■   ☐

STATEMENT REGARDING THE USE OF SCREENING TOOLS. The American College of Obstetricians and Gynecologists (ACOG), through the Committee on Quality Assessment, develops Screening Tools to assist in retrospective chart review to evaluate quality of patient care. They are based primarily on ACOG publications and consensus opinions and do not necessarily mention all acceptable clinical approaches. Departments of obstetrics and gynecology may modify these criteria to reflect local practice. The purpose of Screening Tools is to aid in identifying practice variances that might indicate the need for further review, documentation, or justification. Only peer review can determine whether such variations are appropriate. The use of Screening Tools alone for utilization review or as the basis to deny reimbursement for health services is inappropriate. It is important to understand that Screening Tools are particularly useful in screening cases of morbidity and mortality. However, Screening Tools that address procedures or diagnoses lack specificity or sensitivity, or both; consequently, their usefulness is limited. In using Screening Tools that address procedures or diagnoses, many charts fail the screen, but relatively few, after physician review, are determined to represent quality issues.

ACOG SCREENING TOOL

MYOMECTOMY

STATEMENT REGARDING THE USE OF SCREENING TOOLS. The American College of Obstetricians and Gynecologists (ACOG), through the Committee on Quality Assessment, develops Screening Tools to assist in retrospective chart review to evaluate quality of patient care. They are based primarily on ACOG publications and consensus opinions and do not necessarily mention all acceptable clinical approaches. Departments of obstetrics and gynecology may modify these criteria to reflect local practice. The purpose of Screening Tools is to aid in identifying practice variances that might indicate the need for further review, documentation, or justification. Only peer review can determine whether such variations are appropriate. The use of Screening Tools alone for utilization review or as the basis to deny reimbursement for health services is inappropriate.

It is important to understand that Screening Tools are particularly useful in screening cases of morbidity and mortality. However, Screening Tools that address procedures or diagnoses lack specificity or sensitivity, or both; consequently, their usefulness is limited. In using Screening Tools that address procedures or diagnoses, many charts fail the screen, but relatively few, after physician review, are determined to represent quality issues.

Purpose

The purpose of this Screening Tool is to identify those cases that may require physician review because they fail to meet the listed criteria for screening patients who are undergoing myomectomy and desire to retain uterus. Identified cases may require physician review for QI purposes.

Procedure

Myomectomy (68.29) (**CPT* Codes 58140** [abdominal approach], **58145** [vaginal approach]), or **58551** [laparoscopy with removal of leiomyomata]

Indication

Leiomyomata (ICD-9-CM Codes 218.0–218.9) for patients desiring to retain uterus

Bibliography

American College of Obstetricians and Gynecologists. Surgical alternatives to hysterectomy in the management of leiomyomas. ACOG Practice Bulletin 16. Washington, DC: ACOG, 2000

*CPT only © 1999 American Medical Association. All rights reserved.

Screening Criteria

Myomectomy

Unless otherwise indicated, any time an unshaded box is checked, the chart should be referred for physician review.

Were the following documented in the medical record? Yes No

1. Patient history of either (a *or* b *or* c): ■ ❏
   a. Leiomyomata enlarging the uterus to a size of 12 weeks or greater gestation and are a concern to the patient
   b. Leiomyomata as probable cause of excessive uterine bleeding evidenced by either (1 *or* 2):
      (1) History of excessive uterine bleeding evidenced by profuse bleeding lasting more than 7 days or repetitive periods at less than 21-day intervals
      (2) Anemia due to acute or chronic blood loss
   c. Pelvic discomfort caused by myomata (1 *or* 2 *or* 3)
      (1) Chronic lower abdominal, pelvic, or low back pressure
      (2) Bladder dysfunction not due to urinary tract disorder or disease
      (3) Rectal pressure and bowel dysfunction not related to bowel disorder or disease

2. Prior to the procedure:
   a. Nonmalignant cervical cytology ■ ❏
   b. Anovulation eliminated as cause of abnormal uterine bleeding, if present ■ ❏
   c. When abnormal bleeding is present with ovulatory cycles, assessment for submucous fibroid by dilation and curettage, hysteroscopy, or imaging technique and hysterosalpingography as indicated ■ ❏
   d. Documented discussion of the advantages and disadvantages of myomectomy versus hysterectomy ■ ❏
   e. Negative preoperative pregnancy test result unless patient is postmenopausal ■ ❏

STATEMENT REGARDING THE USE OF SCREENING TOOLS. The American College of Obstetricians and Gynecologists (ACOG), through the Committee on Quality Assessment, develops Screening Tools to assist in retrospective chart review to evaluate quality of patient care. They are based primarily on ACOG publications and consensus opinions and do not necessarily mention all acceptable clinical approaches. Departments of obstetrics and gynecology may modify these criteria to reflect local practice. The purpose of Screening Tools is to aid in identifying practice variances that might indicate the need for further review, documentation, or justification. Only peer review can determine whether such variations are appropriate. The use of Screening Tools alone for utilization review or as the basis to deny reimbursement for health services is inappropriate. It is important to understand that Screening Tools are particularly useful in screening cases of morbidity and mortality. However, Screening Tools that address procedures or diagnoses lack specificity or sensitivity, or both; consequently, their usefulness is limited. In using Screening Tools that address procedures or diagnoses, many charts fail the screen, but relatively few, after physician review, are determined to represent quality issues.

ACOG Screening Tool

Surgery for Genuine Stress Urinary Incontinence

STATEMENT REGARDING THE USE OF SCREENING TOOLS. The American College of Obstetricians and Gynecologists (ACOG), through the Committee on Quality Assessment, develops Screening Tools to assist in retrospective chart review to evaluate quality of patient care. They are based primarily on ACOG publications and consensus opinions and do not necessarily mention all acceptable clinical approaches. Departments of obstetrics and gynecology may modify these criteria to reflect local practice. The purpose of Screening Tools is to aid in identifying practice variances that might indicate the need for further review, documentation, or justification. Only peer review can determine whether such variations are appropriate. The use of Screening Tools alone for utilization review or as the basis to deny reimbursement for health services is inappropriate.

It is important to understand that Screening Tools are particularly useful in screening cases of morbidity and mortality. However, Screening Tools that address procedures or diagnoses lack specificity or sensitivity, or both; consequently, their usefulness is limited. In using Screening Tools that address procedures or diagnoses, many charts fail the screen, but relatively few, after physician review, are determined to represent quality issues.

Purpose

The purpose of this Screening Tool is to identify those cases that may require physician review because they fail to meet the listed criteria for screening patients undergoing surgery for genuine stress urinary incontinence resulting from urethral hypermobility. Identified cases may require physician review for QI purposes.

Procedures

Surgery for genuine stress urinary incontinence (GSUI)*
1. Retropubic procedures (**CPT† Code 58140**)
2. Needle suspension only (**CPT Code 51845** or **57289**)
3. Suburethral plication (**CPT Code 57220**)
4. Paravaginal repair (**CPT Code 57284**)
5. Sling procedures (**CPT Code 57288**)
6. Unspecified procedures for urinary incontinence (**CPT Code 53899**)

Indication

Simple (pure) genuine stress urinary incontinence (ICD-9-CM Code 625.6)

Bibliography

American College of Obstetricians and Gynecologists. Urinary incontinence. ACOG Technical Bulletin 213. Washington, DC: ACOG, 1995

---

* This Screening Tool does not apply to patients who have had either previous surgery for genuine stress urinary incontinence or radical pelvic surgery. These patients may require additional preoperative evaluation.

†CPT only © 1999 American Medical Association. All rights reserved.

Screening Criteria

Surgery for Genuine Stress Urinary Incontinence

Unless otherwise indicated, any time an unshaded box is checked, the chart should be referred for physician review.

Were the following documented in the medical record?	Yes	No
1. Patient history of		
a. Involuntary loss of urine with exertion	■	❏
b. Identification and treatment of transient causes of urinary incontinence, if present (eg, delirium, infection, pharmaceutical causes, psychologic causes, excessive urine production, restricted mobility, and stool impaction)	■	❏
c. Involuntary loss of urine on examination during stress (provocative test with direct visualization of urine loss) and low or absent postvoid residual	■	❏
2. Patient's voiding habits	■	❏
3. Physical or laboratory examination evidence of either (a *or* b)	■	❏
a. Urethral hypermobility		
b. Intrinsic sphincter deficiency		
4. Negative preoperative pregnancy test result unless patient is postmenopausal	■	❏
5. Patient counseled regarding alternative therapy (eg, bladder training, pelvic floor exercises, medications, pessaries, and electrical stimulation)	■	❏

STATEMENT REGARDING THE USE OF SCREENING TOOLS. The American College of Obstetricians and Gynecologists (ACOG), through the Committee on Quality Assessment, develops Screening Tools to assist in retrospective chart review to evaluate quality of patient care. They are based primarily on ACOG publications and consensus opinions and do not necessarily mention all acceptable clinical approaches. Departments of obstetrics and gynecology may modify these criteria to reflect local practice. The purpose of Screening Tools is to aid in identifying practice variances that might indicate the need for further review, documentation, or justification. Only peer review can determine whether such variations are appropriate. The use of Screening Tools alone for utilization review or as the basis to deny reimbursement for health services is inappropriate. It is important to understand that Screening Tools are particularly useful in screening cases of morbidity and mortality. However, Screening Tools that address procedures or diagnoses lack specificity or sensitivity, or both; consequently, their usefulness is limited. In using Screening Tools that address procedures or diagnoses, many charts fail the screen, but relatively few, after physician review, are determined to represent quality issues.

GLOSSARY

Action plan: The product of the root-cause analysis that identifies the strategies that an organization intends to implement to reduce the risk of similar events occurring in the future. The plan should address responsibility for implementation, oversight, pilot testing as appropriate, timelines, and strategies for measuring the effectiveness of the actions.

Benchmark: 1. A point of reference or standard by which something can be measured, compared, or judged, as in benchmarks of performance. 2. A standard unit for the basis of comparison, that is, a universal unit that is identified with sufficient detail so that other similar classifications can be compared as being above, below, or comparable to the benchmark.

Clinical pathway: A treatment regimen, agreed on by consensus, that includes all the elements of care, regardless of the effect on patient outcomes. It is a broader look at care and may include tests and X-rays that do not affect patient recovery. *Synonyms:* clinical path, critical pathway.

Continuous Quality Improvement: A set of techniques for continuous study and improvement of the processes of delivering health care services and products to meet the needs and expectations of the customers of those services and products. It has three basic elements: 1) customer knowledge, 2) a focus on processes of health care delivery, and 3) statistical approaches that aim to reduce variations in those processes.

Credentialing: The process of obtaining, verifying, and assessing the qualifications of a health care practitioner to provide patient care services in or for a health care organization. The determination is based on an evaluation of the individual's current license, education, training, experience, competence, and professional judgment. The process is the basis for making appointments to the professional staff of the health care organization. The process also provides information for granting clinical privileges to licensed independent practitioners.

Disruptive behavior: An aberrant style of personal interaction with physicians, hospital personnel, patients, family members, or others that potentially interferes with patient care.

Facilitator: In quality improvement, a person who has developed special expertise in the QI process. He or she does not belong to a QI team but helps it achieve results by helping to focus its efforts, teaching QI methods, consulting with the team leader, and helping connect the work to the knowledge necessary for improvement.

Indicator: 1. A measure used to determine, over time, performance of functions, processes, and outcomes. 2. A statistical value that provides an indication of the condition or direction, over time, of performance of a defined process or achievement of a defined outcome.

Medical review criteria: Systematically developed statements that can be used to assess specific health care decisions, services, and outcomes.

Outcome: Denotes the effects of care on the health status of patients and populations. Improvements in the patient's knowledge and salutary changes in the patient's behavior are included under a broad definition of health status, and so is the degree of the patient's satisfaction with care.

Outliers: 1. Any measurement that is beyond a predetermined threshold of appropriate care. 2. Health care providers with performance or outcomes rates that are outside the range of expected rates after adjustment for patient or other characteristics.

Performance measures: Methods or instruments to estimate or monitor the extent to which the actions of a health care practitioner or provider conform to the clinical practice guideline.

Physician impairment: The inability of a physician to practice medicine with reasonable skill and with safety to patients due to a disability, such as alcohol or drug abuse, mental illness, handicap, or senility.

Plan–Do–Study–Act (PDSA) cycle: A four-part method for discovering and correcting assignable causes to improve the quality of processes. Modification of the Plan–Do–Check–Act cycle. *Synonyms:* Deming cycle; Shewhart cycle.

Practice guidelines: Systematically developed statements to assist practitioner and patient decisions about appropriate health care for specific clinical circumstances.

Preceptorship: An educational program designed to give the professionally trained students experience outside the academic environment working in the specialty area of their choice with a physician or other advisory supervisors.

Privileging: The process whereby a specific scope and content of patient care services (that is, clinical privileges) are authorized for a health care practitioner by a health care organization based on evaluation of the individual's credentials and performance.

Proctoring: Observation and evaluation of a practitioner for appointment or clinical privileges.

Process: Denotes what is actually done in giving and receiving care. It includes the patient's activities in seeking care and carrying it out as well as the practitioner's activities in making a diagnosis and recommending or implementing treatment.

Quality improvement: The attainment, or process of attaining, a new level of performance or quality that is superior to any previous level of quality.

Recredentialing: The process of determining and certifying the competence of a physician or other professional at some time after the initial determination of his or her qualification for licensure or hospital privileges. Recredentialing is required at periodic intervals (such as every 2 years) in most hospitals and other types of health care organizations. Recredentialing focuses on physicians' actual performance, rather than on physicians' capacity to perform well, as reflected, for example, in passing a written examination.

Root-cause analysis: A process for identifying the basic or causal factor(s) that underlie variation in performance, including the occurrence or possible occurrence of a sentinel event.

Sentinel event: An unexpected occurrence or variation involving death or serious physical or psychologic injury, or risk thereof. Serious injury specifically includes loss of limb or function. The event is called "sentinel" because it sends a signal or sounds a warning that requires immediate attention.

Structure: Denotes the attributes of the settings in which care occurs. This includes the attributes of material resources (such as facilities, equipment, and money), of human resources (such as the number and qualifications of personnel), and of organizational structure (such as medical staff organization, methods of peer review, and methods of reimbursement).

REFERENCES

1. Lohr KN, ed. Medicare: a strategy for quality assurance. Washington, DC: National Academy Press, 1990

2. Berwick DM. Charting the future of healthcare improvement. Qual Lett Healthc Lead 1998;10:2–4

3. Gaucher EJ, Coffey RJ. Integrating total quality management and quality assurance. In: Total quality in healthcare: from theory to practice. San Francisco: Jossey-Bass Publishers, 1993:54–77

4. Berwick DM. Continuous improvement as an ideal in health care. N Engl J Med 1989;320:53–56

5. Zinberg S. Stratification and standards: a quality assurance perspective. Presidential Address. Am J Obstet Gynecol 1991;164:722–728

6. Palmer RH, Banks NJ. Designing and testing medical review criteria and performance measures. In: Schoenbaum SC, Sundwall DN, Bergman D, Buckle JM, Chernov A, George J, et al. Using clinical practice guidelines to evaluate quality of care. Rockville, Maryland: Agency for Health Care Policy and Research, U.S. Department of Health and Human Services, Public Health Service, 1995 March; AHCPR publication no. 95-0045:31–71

7. Donabedian A. The quality of care. How can it be assessed? JAMA 1988;260:1743–1748

8. Parsons ML, Purdon TF, Craig B. Restructured quality and utilization management. In: Parsons ML, Murdaugh CL, Purdon TF, Jarrell BE. Guide to clinical resource management. Gaithersburg, Maryland: Aspen Publishers, 1997: 16–33

9. McEachern E, Lord JT. The role of physicians in prioritizing the work of teams and the organization. In: Burton R. The physician leader's guide, 2nd edition. Alexandria, Virginia: Capitol Publications, 1998:27–40

10. Joint Commission on Accreditation of Healthcare Organizations. Improving organization performance. In: Comprehensive accreditation manual for hospitals: the official handbook. Oakbrook Terrace, Illinois: JCAHO, 2000: PI-1–PI-34

11. Campion P. Clinical practice guideline development "tool kit." Orlando, Florida: IHI Forum, 1997

12. Schoenbaum SC, Sundwall DN, Bergman D, Buckle JM, Chernov A, George J, et al. Using clinical practice guidelines to evaluate quality of care. Rockville, Maryland: Agency for Health Care Policy and Research, U.S. Department of Health and Human Services, Public Health Service, 1995 March; AHCPR publication no. 95-0045:9–13

13. Darby M. 12 ways to get physician buy-in to practice guidelines. Qual Lett Healthc Lead 1998;10(3):2–3

14. Kotter JP. Leading change. Boston: Harvard Business School Pr, 1996:25–30

15. Juran D. Achieving sustained quantifiable results in an interdepartmental quality improvement project. Jt Comm J Qual Improv 1994;20:105–119

16. Berwick DM, Godfrey AB, Roessner J. Using the scientific method to define problems. In: Curing health care: new strategies for quality improvement. San Francisco: Jossey–Bass Publishers, 1990:46–66

17. Take the lead out of quality improvement projects. Hosp Peer Rev 1996;21:19–20, 33–34

18. Berwick DM, Godfrey AB, Roessner J. Resource C: three project reports. In: Curing health care: new strategies for

quality improvement. San Francisco: Jossey–Bass Publishers, 1990:221–274

19. Flamm B, Kabcenell A, Berwick D, Roessner J. A step-by-step guide to reducing cesarean section rates. In: Reducing cesarean section rates while maintaining maternal and infant outcomes. Boston: Institute for Healthcare Improvement, 1997:13–35

20. Laffel G, Blumenthal D. The case for using industrial quality management science in health care organizations. JAMA 1989;262:2869–2873

21. Hyde GL, Miscall BG. The impaired surgeon: diagnosis, treatment, and reentry. Chicago, Illinois: American College of Surgeons, 1995

22. Stevens, S. Disruptive doctors exert a devastating and demoralizing impact on practices. Physicians Financ News 1997;15(3):1, 34–35

23. Joint Commission on Accreditation of Healthcare Organizations. Accreditation Committee approves exam-ples of voluntary reportable sentinel events. Sentinel Event Alert; issue 4. Oakbrook Terrace, Illinois: JCAHO, 1999

24. Joint Commission on Accreditation of Healthcare Organizations. Comprehensive accreditation manual for hospitals: the official handbook. Oakbrook Terrace, Illinois: JCAHO, 2000:SE-1–SE-8

25. American Academy of Family Physicians, American College of Obstetricians and Gynecologists. Recommended Core Educational Guidelines for Family Practice Residents: Maternity and Gynecologic Care. AAFP-ACOG Policy Statement 73. Kansas City, Missouri: AAFP; Washington, DC: ACOG, 1998

26. American Academy of Family Physicians, American College of Obstetricians and Gynecologists. Joint Statement on Cooperative Practice and Hospital Privileges. AAFP-ACOG Policy Statement 73. Kansas City, Missouri: AAFP; Washington, DC: ACOG, 1998

APPENDIXES

Appendix A. Sample Data Collection Form: Department Gynecology Statistics

	Year _____		Year _____	
	Inpatient	Outpatient	Inpatient	Outpatient
Total surgical procedures				
Gynecologic deaths				
Same admission—unplanned return to OR				
Admission after ambulatory surgery				
Unplanned readmissions within 14 days				
Minor procedures				
D&C (not related to pregnancy) (ICD-9-CM Procedural Codes 69.09)				
Hysteroscopies				
Diagnostic (68.12)				
Operative (68.16, 68.21–23, 68.29)				
Total laparoscopies				
Diagnostic (54.21)				
Operative (68.15, 68.16)				
For sterilization (66.21, 66.22, 66.29)				
Cervical cerclage (67.5)				
Laser or cold knife conizations (67.2)				
Loop excisions of the transformation zone (LETZ) (67.32)				
Major procedures				
Hysterectomies (68.3, 68.4)				
Abdominal (68.9)				
Vaginal (68.5, 68.59, 68.9)				
Laparoscopically assisted (68.51)				
Exploratory laparotomies (54.1, 54.11, 54.12)				
Operations for stress incontinence (59.3–59.7)				
Abdominal (59.5, 59.6, 59.71)				
Vaginal (59.3, 59.4, 59.72, 59.79)				
Radical surgery (68.6, 68.7, 68.8)				

Abbreviations: OR indicates operating room; D&C, dilation and curettage.

Appendix B. Sample Data Collection Form: Department Obstetric Statistics

	Year _____		Year _____	
	Number	Percent	Number	Percent
Obstetric admissions (or discharges)				
Mothers delivered				
Vaginal				
Abdominal (total cesarean)* (ICD-9-CM Procedural Codes 74.0, 74.1, 74.2, 74.4, 74.99)				
Primary* cesarean deliveries†				
Repeat‡ cesarean deliveries§				
High-risk pregnancies				
Pregnancy-induced hypertension				
Diabetes				
Third-trimester bleeding				
Substance abuse				
Multiple gestation				
Other				
Induction of labor (oxytocin/AROM)‖ (74.01, 73.09, 73.1, 73.4)				
Augmentation of labor				
Anesthesia for delivery				
None				
Perineal				
Conduction (spinal, epidural)				
General				
Epidural for labor#				
Previous cesarean deliveries				
Elective repeat				
Trial of labor; repeat cesareans				
Trial of labor; vaginal delivery**				
Maternal deaths				

	Year _____		Year _____	
	Number	Percent	Number	Percent
Maternal transfers				
In				
Out				
Births				
Cephalic presentation				
Forceps/vacuum (72.0–72.4, 72.7–72.9)				
Cesarean delivery				
Breech presentation				
Vaginal birth (72.5–72.6)				
Cesarean delivery				
Apgar scores < 5 at 5 minutes				
Neonatal transfers				
In				
Out				

* $\dfrac{\text{No. of cesarean deliveries}}{\text{No. of live births}} \times 100$

† $\dfrac{\text{No. of primary cesarean deliveries}}{\text{No. of live births minus total No. of previous cesareans}} \times 100$

‡The term "repeat" refers to this delivery and the previous delivery(-ies).

§ $\dfrac{\text{No. of repeat cesarean deliveries}}{\text{Total No. of cesarean deliveries}} \times 100$

‖ $\dfrac{\text{No. of women induced}}{\text{No. of women in labor}} \times 100$

$\dfrac{\text{No. of epidurals}}{\text{No. of women in labor}} \times 100$

** $\dfrac{\text{No. of VBACs}}{\text{No. of previous cesarean deliveries}} \times 100$

Appendix C.

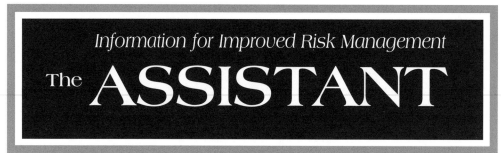

Information for Improved Risk Management

Number 4

The **ASSISTANT**

Department of
Professional
Liability

Informed Consent

Informed consent is a legal doctrine that requires a physician to obtain consent to render treatment, to perform an operation, or to carry out many diagnostic procedures. Without informed consent the physician may be held liable for violation of the patient's rights, even when the treatment was appropriate and rendered with due care. It is inappropriate for a physician to provide medical care to an individual without that individual granting either expressed or implied permission for the physician to act. A person must give permission for any intentional "touching" of his or her person by another; without permission, such contact is "battery."

Informed consent is a process, not a form. Consent often is equated with the document a patient signs in agreement to a procedure or treatment her physician believes to be advisable or necessary. Although some form of documentation is necessary for purposes of treatment and legal defense, a consent form cannot replace the exchange of information between the physician and the patient that culminates in the patient accepting or refusing a specific procedure or treatment. The document is intended to record this process.

Effective informed consent requires active participation by both the physician and the patient. The patient must provide accurate and complete information to the physician and, if matters are unclear, ask questions. The physician must ensure that the patient has sufficient information about the treatment or procedure to give valid informed consent. There are many tools that the physician can use to assist in the informed consent process, such as education pamphlets, videos, and interactive computer programs.

The physician should allow the patient reasonable time to contemplate all the information given and should encourage questions to ensure that the patient fully understands the information provided. Physicians should inform their patients of medically appropriate treatment options regardless of their cost or the extent to which the treatment options are covered by health insurance plans.

The laws governing informed consent vary from state to state, and physicians should acquaint themselves with the law in their respective states. In most states, the law makes informed consent a nondelegable duty of the treating or performing physician. The courts have developed two standards for determining the adequacy of the informed consent process. Many states still use the reasonable physician standard. This standard of disclosure is measured by what is customary practice in the medical community for physicians to divulge to patients. In recent years, however, the majority of jurisdictions have preferred to accept the reasonable patient standard. Under the reasonable patient standard, disclosure of information is based on what a reasonable person in the patient's position would want to know in similar circumstances. This standard is based on the patient's perception rather than on professional perception of what the patient should know.

Generally, in jurisdictions that follow the professional or reasonable physician standard, less information needs to be revealed than in those jurisdictions that adhere to the reasonable patient standard. For example, if a risk of a procedure or treatment is extremely remote but may have serious consequences to the patient, the risk should be disclosed under the reasonable patient standard, but it may not have to be disclosed under the reasonable physician standard.

Although legislation in some states may set particular standards for disclosure of specific information, a physician should keep in mind that, to obtain fully informed consent, he or she must explain to the patient

- The diagnosis and the nature of the condition or illness calling for medical intervention
- The nature and purpose of the treatment or procedure recommended
- The material risks and potential complications associated with the recommended treatment or procedure
- The feasible alternative treatments or procedures, including the option of taking no action, with a description of material risks and potential complications associated with choosing the alternatives or no action
- The relative probability of success for the treatment or procedure in understandable terms

No result should ever be guaranteed to the patient.

Consent is "fully informed" only when the patient knows and understands the information necessary to make an informed decision about a treatment or procedure. Notations to the patient's file should be as complete as possible. These notations should include that the informed consent discussion took place, risks and benefits were fully explained, the patient had an opportunity to ask questions, and the patient consented to the treatment or procedure.

There is no informed consent if the treatment or procedure extends beyond the scope of consent. If the care or the risks associated with the care are substantially different than that contemplated by the patient, then the courts may find that the original informed consent was not sufficient.

There are certain circumstances for which special informed consent rules apply. These are emergencies, situations involving minors, and those rare circumstances where authorization for a treatment or procedure is obtained from a court.

In a medical emergency, the physician might treat a patient without obtaining the patient's prior consent to the treatment or procedure. For the event to be considered a genuine emergency, however, 1) the patient must be unconscious or incapacitated and 2) suffering from a life-threatening or serious health-threatening situation requiring immediate medical attention. Because the patient is unable to consent in these instances, consent is implied. This is based on the theory that if the patient was competent, the patient would have consented to the care rendered.

Because emergencies present unique situations, it is particularly important for the physician to document in the patient's record the reason the care was rendered. This should include a chronological description of the event, the objective indications of the emergency, a description of the patient's condition at the time of the emergency, an explanation as to why immediate medical attention was necessary, and a description of attempts to obtain consent from the patient and other responsible parties.

Special informed consent rules applicable to minors vary widely from state to state. Basically, minors are unable to consent to medical treatment unless they are "emancipated" by virtue of living apart from their parents and by being financially self-supporting, married, or in the military. If a minor is not emancipated, physicians must obtain consent from the minor's parent or legal guardian when providing all but emergency care. All states, however, have enacted at least one statute modifying this rule in a variety of ways. These statutes usually establish criteria or circumstances under which a minor is permitted to consent to medical care without parental permission.

Most of these statutes set a statutory age of consent or allow minors to consent in the case of contraception, pregnancy, drug and alcohol abuse, or the treatment of sexually transmissible infections. It is important for physicians to know the law in their state. To find out more about state-specific requirements, physicians should contact their state medical society. As with all patients, a minor should be fully informed before medical treatment is provided.

Physicians also may be confronted with situations in which a patient has refused medical treatment. A patient who is informed of the material risks and benefits of a particular treatment or procedure may elect to forego that treatment or procedure, despite a physician's medical recommendation. It is not uncommon for such decisions to be made because of personal preference, comfort, or economic reasons. In these circumstances, a physician should document the informed refusal in the patient's medical record. It should be noted in the record that the physician recommended a particular treatment or procedure to the patient, the material risks and benefits of the treatment or procedure were explained to the patient, and the patient refused the treatment or procedure. If the refusal for medical treatment is truly informed and the refusal is documented, a physician should be protected in the event of a medical malpractice lawsuit stemming from the consequences of the refusal.

Emerging issues regarding informed consent in some jurisdictions include the physician's responsibility to disclose his or her financial interests or incentives in managed health care plans and the physician's responsibility to disclose his or her experience and skill level in performing a procedure or treatment. Individual state medical societies can provide up-to-date information on these issues.

For further information, refer to the ACOG Committee Opinion Number 108, "Ethical Dimensions of Informed Consent."

For more information on this and other professional liability issues, call the Department of Professional Liability, (202) 863-2582. For a risk assessment checklist on professional liability insurance issues, please see *Office Risk Management Check-up* No. 4, "Informed Consent."

The information in this monograph should not be construed as legal advice. As always, physicians should consult their personal attorneys about legal requirements in their jurisdiction and for legal advice on a particular matter.

Copyright ©1998 The American College of Obstetricians and Gynecologists
Department of Professional Liability
409 12th Street, SW, PO Box 96920, Washington, DC 20090-6920

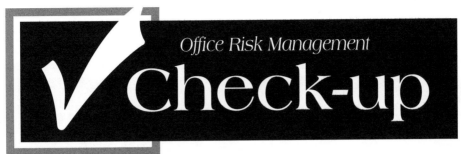

Office Risk Management

Check-up

Number 4

Department of
Professional
Liability

Informed Consent

1. Can you be held liable for violating a patient's rights if you do not advise the patient of the risks and benefits of the treatment or procedure?   Yes ☐   No ☐

2. Does a patient have a valid claim against you if you provide nonemergency medical care to her without obtaining her prior permission?   Yes ☐   No ☐

3. Do you set aside time to allow a patient to ask you questions as part of the informed consent process?   Yes ☐   No ☐

4. Do you inform your patients of medically appropriate treatment options even if those options are costly or not covered by insurance?   Yes ☐   No ☐

5. Are you familiar with the general and specific laws in your state governing informed consent?   Yes ☐   No ☐

6. Do you know if your state uses the reasonable physician standard or the reasonable patient standard?   Yes ☐   No ☐

7. Do you provide notations or some other form of documentation to the patient's file detailing the informed consent discussion?   Yes ☐   No ☐

8. Do you know the emergency circumstances that allow you to treat a patient without her prior consent?   Yes ☐   No ☐

9. Are you familiar with the rules of your state pertaining to informed consent for minors?   Yes ☐   No ☐

10. Do you have an office protocol to document a patient's informed refusal of a recommended treatment or procedure?   Yes ☐   No ☐

For more information on this and other professional liability issues, call the Department of Professional Liability, (202) 863-2582. For a detailed monograph of these informed consent issues, please see *The Assistant* No. 4, "Informed Consent."

Copyright © 1998 The American College of Obstetricians and Gynecologists
Department of Professional Liability
409 12th Street, SW, PO Box 96920, Washington, DC 20090-6920

Appendix D.

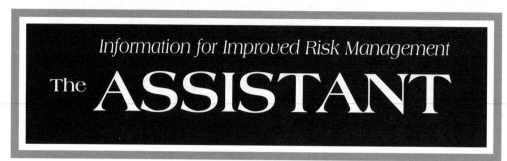

Information for Improved Risk Management

The **ASSISTANT**

Number 5

Department of Professional Liability

Informed Consent Forms

Informed consent is a process, not a form. A written consent form cannot replace the exchange of information between you and your patient.

In some states, a signed consent form creates a rebuttable presumption of a valid informed consent on the part of the patient if it meets certain criteria. In states without this type of legislation, a consent form is just one piece of evidence for the defense in a case alleging lack of informed consent.

A consent form should incorporate the elements of the informed consent conversation relayed in nontechnical language. The form should include a description of each procedure, its risks and expected benefits, its alternatives, and the risks of no treatment. It should be signed by the patient in the presence of an attesting witness. A blanket consent form will usually be found insufficient to prove the content of the informed consent discussion.

Regardless of whether consent was obtained during your patient's office visit, another consent process may occur in the hospital setting, and special considerations of that setting may affect the manner in which the consent is obtained. It is your responsi-

bility, not that of the hospital, to provide the necessary information to the patient and obtain informed consent. The hospital, however, may be liable for failing to intervene when it has knowledge that a procedure is being performed without proper consent. When a hospital follows the policy of having a nurse or ward clerk obtain a patient's signature on a consent form, it is at this time that a patient may indicate uncertainty or lack of understanding. Once a hospital staff member becomes aware of the patient's confusion, the staff member should notify the physician responsible for that patient.

You should not delegate the task of resolving doubts or answering the patient's questions, because you might be held liable for failure to obtain valid informed consent if the patient agrees to a procedure based on the misinformation provided by another staff member. There must exist some evidence of consent—oral or written, expressed or implied—granting authority for you to proceed, or evidence of circumstances in which consent could not be obtained (eg, in emergency care situations).

For more information on this and other professional liability issues, call the Department of Professional Liability, (202) 863-2582. For a risk assessment checklist on informed consent forms, please see *Office Risk Management Check-up* No. 5, "Informed Consent Forms."

The information in this monograph should not be construed as legal advice. As always, physicians should consult their personal attorneys about legal requirements in their jurisdiction and for legal advice on a particular matter.

Copyright © 1998 The American College of Obstetricians and Gynecologists
Department of Professional Liability
409 12th Street, SW, PO Box 96920, Washington, DC 20090-6920

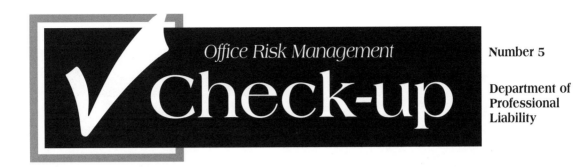

Informed Consent Forms

1. Are you familiar with the requirements in your state regarding written informed consent forms?

   Yes ☐   No ☐

2. Does your consent form incorporate a description of the test/procedure, its risks and expected outcomes, alternatives, and risks of no treatment?

   Yes ☐   No ☐

3. If your patient is going to be hospitalized, have you gone through the informed consent process prior to her hospital admission?

   Yes ☐   No ☐

For more information on this and other professional liability issues, call the Department of Professional Liability, (202) 863-2582. For a detailed monograph of informed consent forms issues, please see *The Assistant* No. 5, "Informed Consent Forms."

Copyright © 1998 The American College of Obstetricians and Gynecologists
Department of Professional Liability
409 12th Street, SW, PO Box 96920, Washington, DC 20090-6920

Appendix E.

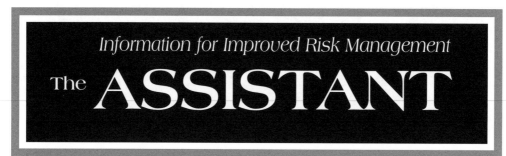

Information for Improved Risk Management

The **ASSISTANT**

Number 10

Department of
Professional
Liability

Risk Management in the Hospital Setting

Most events that lead to claims against a physician take place in the hospital setting. Obstetrician–gynecologists, as surgeons, conduct many of the most frequently performed surgical procedures and, as a result, are exposed to a greater risk of liability than other physicians.

Risk management in the hospital begins prior to admission. It is important for the physician to properly prepare and fully discuss all details of a patient's hospitalization with her. This discussion should include the reason for admission, the procedure recommended, the alternatives, and potential risks and complications. Informed consent discussions, as well as any informed refusal discussions, should be documented in the patient's medical record. Please refer to the issues of *The Assistant* entitled "Informed Consent" and "Informed Consent Forms."

It is vital to convey to your patient the possibility of a complication or change in the expected outcome, because a patient's surprise and disappointment often lead to lawsuits. For example, the patient who experiences fever, infection, or an extended hospital stay following surgery is less likely to sue her physician if she was properly forewarned. In addition, it is necessary to inform a patient of the risk that a procedure (eg, sterilization) may not always be effective. The patient who experiences a complication (including neonatal complications) requires additional time, attention, and information from her physician.

The medical record is an important method of communication. It is essential to examine records for clarity and completeness. A patient's chart should be reviewed before she is examined; this review should include checking orders regularly and verifying the

notes of nurses, other physicians, and residents. For obstetric patients, a risk assessment form or checklist, if used, should be completed and included in the patient's medical record.

The accurate transfer of the patient's record from the office to the hospital is an essential element in risk management. All risk assessment forms must be copied and sent to the hospital prior to the patient's estimated date of arrival. The record of a high-risk patient should be flagged prior to transfer to alert those involved with the patient's care of specific problems that need close attention. Often, upon arrival at the hospital, the patient's record is first reviewed by someone other than the primary physician. Once records of prenatal care are transferred to the hospital, they must be updated to include patient encounters in the office that occurred subsequent to the records transfer.

If a resident is working under your direction, do not merely co-sign a chart and assume it is accurate. It is imperative to read and assess the chart. If you disagree with the evaluation, make a note and point it out to the resident. The rationale behind your decision also should be noted in the chart. This also applies to nurses' notes, ie, are the proper medications and solutions being given and are the amounts accurate? Nurses observe patients and usually communicate their findings through progress notes. Proper observation and evaluation of this prime area of communication will demonstrate that timely and appropriate care has been given.

In a complicated situation, it may be necessary to consult with another physician or refer the patient elsewhere for care. No physician should expect that his or her knowledge is complete and superior in all instances. Courts have little sympathy for situations in which a collaborative approach might have resulted in better care. Timely consultation suggests prudence on the part of the physician. Discuss the situation with the patient prior to the consultation, because an unfamiliar face in the hospital setting may cause unnecessary alarm to the patient and her family. You also should notify the hospital staff if there will be a consulting physician involved and the role that he or she will play. Moreover, it must be made clear who has the main responsibility for the patient, who is in charge, and who can write orders for the patient. Because a number of people can be held liable for an injury, establishing who holds the primary authority for the patient's care can minimize the risk of miscommunication. All staff members need to know who should be consulted when a problem arises.

If the patient's hospitalization occurs as a result of your referral to a physician in another specialty, keep in mind that often you are considered by the patient and others as her primary physician. Never allow a patient to feel abandoned. It is important for her to be aware of the circumstances and to give her consent for the referral. Let the patient know you are concerned and make every effort to monitor her care. Drop in to see her while she is confined in the hospital. Let the other specialist know you want to be kept apprised of her progress, and if surgery is necessary, that you want to be told when it will take place. If a complication should arise, showing interest and maintaining a healthy rapport often can be helpful in preventing a lawsuit.

Hospital rules and protocols are established to ensure a uniform quality of care. In an effort to help prevent patient injury and minimize liability risks, all members of the health care team must clearly understand hospital systems and protocols. A physician's failure to comply with such hospital policies may subsequently be interpreted as a violation of the standard of care. Physicians should know, understand, and comply with these policies.

Physicians who work in hospitals need to be aware that the law recognizes the existence of a vicarious relationship based on the legal concepts of the "borrowed servant" and the "captain of the ship." Under these doctrines, one person might be liable for the acts of an employee of another if the negligent act occurs while that employee is under the first person's direction or control.

The "borrowed servant" rule would apply to the members of the surgical team who were employees of someone other than the surgeon if the surgeon had the opportunity to direct the team during surgery. In this way, the surgeon would be exercising the traditional supervisory role of the employer. A physician also can be held liable for a negligent act that occurred out of the physician's presence when the task involved improper delegation of duties (eg, delegating to unlicensed personnel a task requiring professional judgment).

A surgeon can be held liable under the "captain of the ship" doctrine for the actions of the other members of the surgical team if the surgical personnel are under the supervision or control of the surgeon. Liability might be imposed by virtue of the surgeon's supervisory responsibilities, even though the surgeon in no way aided or encouraged the negligent act. Originally, the term "captain of the ship" was used merely to explain the operation of the borrowed servant doctrine; however, with continuous use, it emerged as a separate doctrine. It is of utmost importance that physicians properly communicate, delegate, and supervise any member of the health care team who might come in contact with a patient in the hospital. Risk management is a team effort. The move toward the employment of more nonphysician clinical personnel has made it necessary for physicians to be aware of the extent of their liability.

Technologic advances have greatly improved patient care but also have contributed to the creation of new areas of risk for the physician as well as elevated expectations on the part of the patient. Keeping informed of new techniques and procedures is a fundamental part of good medicine in the hospital setting. It often is argued that the very existence of certain technology leads to overutilization or unnecessary intervention. It is essential for those who use new advances (eg, laparoscopy, teleradiology) to be properly trained and to understand the mechanics of the technology. Physicians should understand and employ mechanisms for periodic evaluation and testing of equipment in order to anticipate any malfunction. Equipment must be maintained properly and operate reliably. Product liability can lead to physician liability. Hospital policies should provide for a backup and cross-check of every system.

Although gynecologic claims are increasingly more frequent, the largest awards against the specialty occur in obstetric cases involving neurologically impaired infants. Thus, the highest risk area for the obstetrician–gynecologist is the delivery room. Prompt attention to a high-risk situation, proper delegation of responsibilities, and requesting the presence of a pediatrician, neonatologist, or other medical personnel skilled in resuscitation demonstrate good practice. High-risk pregnancies are not always identified prior to delivery. In many instances, a judgment call is necessary. The importance of accurately documenting the situation and the rationale for your decisions cannot be overemphasized.

The widespread use of recording technology in the hospital setting has affected the practice of obstetrics and gynecology. Each hospital should develop guidelines concerning the recording of routine and emergency procedures by health care personnel as well as the recording of deliveries by third parties or family members. These policies should be discussed before the procedure or soon after the physician–patient relationship has been established. Written consent from the patient or guardian and the involved health care personnel should be obtained, and the specific purposes for which the images may be used should be indicated.

Risk management in daily practice can substantially reduce the potential for patient injury and protect physicians against groundless claims. Diligence in practice and special attention to those procedures that carry additional risk help reduce liability problems. Keeping up to date on current literature and technologic advances, maintaining complete records, properly obtaining informed consent, responding to complications in a timely manner, complying with local rules and regulations, and most importantly, developing effective communication skills should be incorporated into everyday practice.

For more information on this and other professional liability issues, call the Department of Professional Liability, (202) 863-2582. For a risk assessment checklist on this issue, please see *Office Risk Management Check-up* No. 10, "Risk Management in the Hospital Setting."

The information in this monograph should not be construed as legal advice. As always, physicians should consult their personal attorneys about legal requirements in their jurisdiction and for legal advice on a particular matter.

Copyright © 1999 by the American College of Obstetricians and Gynecologists. All rights reserved. No part of this publication may be reproduced, stored in a retrieval system, or transmitted, in any form or by any means, electronic, mechanical, photocopying, recording, or otherwise, without prior written permission from the publisher.

Department of Professional Liability
409 12th Street, SW, PO Box 96920, Washington, DC 20090-6920

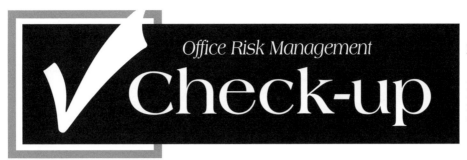

Risk Management in the Hospital Setting

1. Do you discuss the details of your patient's hospitalization with her prior to her admission into the hospital? Yes ☐ No ☐

2. Is the patient's record accurate and up to date when it is transferred to the hospital? Yes ☐ No ☐

3. Are subsequent patient encounters entered into the patient's prenatal record at the hospital? Yes ☐ No ☐

4. If another physician is involved in the care of your patient, have you discussed the circumstances with your patient? Yes ☐ No ☐

5. Are you aware of your hospital's policies and protocols pertaining to the treatment your patient is to receive? Yes ☐ No ☐

6. Have you had the appropriate training for any new technology you intend to use? Yes ☐ No ☐

7. Have you discussed with your patient your institution's policy regarding videotaping procedures? Yes ☐ No ☐

For more information on this and other professional liability issues, call the Department of Professional Liability, (202) 863-2582.

For a detailed monograph on this issue, please see *The Assistant* No. 10, "Risk Management in the Hospital Setting."

Copyright © 1999 by the American College of Obstetricians and Gynecologists. All rights reserved. No part of this publication may be reproduced, stored in a retrieval system, or transmitted, in any form or by any means, electronic, mechanical, photocopying, recording, or otherwise, without prior written permission from the publisher.

Department of Professional Liability
409 12th Street, SW, PO Box 96920, Washington, DC 20090-6920